Migrant Nurses

Motivation, integration and contribution

Andrea Winkelmann-Gleed

Forewords by
Roswyn Hakesley-Brown
and
Barbara L Nichols

Radcliffe Publishing
Oxford • Seattle

Radcliffe Publishing Ltd
18 Marcham Road
Abingdon
Oxon OX14 1AA
United Kingdom

www.radcliffe-oxford.com
Electronic catalogue and worldwide online ordering facility.

British Library Cataloguing in Publication Data

A catalogue record for this book is available from the British Library.

ISBN-10 1 84619 007 X
ISBN-13 978 1 84619 007 0

Typeset by Aarontype Ltd, Easton, Bristol
Printed and bound by TJ International Ltd, Padstow, Cornwall

Contents

Foreword

International migration is nothing new. It has been around for centuries. There have usually been major political or personal imperatives which have caused individuals or communities to leave everything behind and undertake long, often perilous journeys to new domiciles in alien and unfamiliar environments. It was ever thus.

What is new is today's migration diaspora, which presents radically different challenges to those historically documented. This is particularly so when globalisation, the knowledge explosion and increasing polarisation between the developing and developed world are added to the mix.

Andrea Winkelmann-Gleed has taken on this complexity by providing robust, empirical evidence and a forensic analysis of migration in relation to a particular occupational community, that of migrant nurses.

Her valuable contribution to the literature is particularly timely, in view of the increasing worldwide shortage of nurses, which constitutes an emerging global crisis. This is the first text to offer a comprehensive analysis of the motivation, integration and positive contribution that migrant nurses can make to healthcare in the UK. It offers unique insights essential for using this significant element of the healthcare workforce in an intelligent, balanced and just manner.

This book has the potential to provide a crucial fulcrum for informing debate and the shape of future professional and political policy in relation to the more efficient utilisation of all nurse migrants. This includes not only those who are part of planned overseas recruitment exercises but also those who constitute a previously untapped nursing workforce who are already in the UK. These are migrant nurses who are also refugees.

At an operational level, much can be gained from this text to inform the development of strategies which invest in the creation of a multicultural workforce, with the corresponding organisational infrastructure to support this.

The author wisely recognises that capitalising on the skills of migrant nurses is not without its challenges. However, we know that migrating nurses have 'get up and go'. The evidence demonstrates that they do it for a variety of reasons. We cannot afford to ignore or talk down the richness that they can bring to healthcare in the UK. To do this, we must not only be able to work smart, but be visionary in using these windows of *migration opportunity*. It is worth remembering Nelson Mandela's salutary exhortation:

> Action without vision is merely dreaming. Vision without action is just passing the time of day. Put the two together and you can change the world.

This book will help us to do just that.

Roswyn Hakesley-Brown
Chair, Refugee Nurses Task Force
December 2005

Foreword

Mobility is a fact of modern life, and nurse migrants play an essential role in today's global healthcare economy. *Migrant Nurses: Motivation, integration and contribution* is a book documenting the impact of nurse migration as a worldwide shortage of nurses emerges. Although the book describes the experience of migrant nurses in Britain, it is a fascinating collection of personal stories that illuminates the larger professional and socio-political forces driving global nurse migration.

Confronting a range of topics, such as cultural and ethnic differences, ethical issues, integration into the workforce, motivation to migrate, and contributions of migrant nurses, the author offers a focused look at the economics of healthcare shaped by migrant nurses. The personal stories identify the vulnerability of migrant nurses to factors such as racism, sexism and harassment. The analysis of issues identifies that, embedded within the phenomenon of migration are multiple degrading relationships with peers, subordinates, superiors and other health workers that are reinforced by stereotypes of race, ethnicity, and low tolerance for difference.

The personal stories also magnify the scope and complexity of nurse migration and its importance to the delivery of care and to national health systems.

In a globalized and exceedingly mobile world, the key questions raised and the challenges identified make this book important reading for our times.

Barbara L Nichols, DHL, MS, RN, FAAN
Chief Executive Officer
Commission on Graduates of Foreign Nursing Schools
Philadelphia, Pennsylvania USA
December 2005

Preface

My interest in the issues of international migration and the sharing of skills extends back to having worked with poor communities and refugee groups in Southern Sudan, Djibouti, Somalia, Ethiopia and Rwandan refugees camps in Tanzania. Furthermore, field research in Cambodia and life in multicultural parts of Germany and the UK taught me that social exclusion is multifaceted and not just exercised by majorities towards minorities and those who are 'different'. There are hidden facets to exclusion, institutional aspects, prejudices within and among minority groups and we are all guilty at times of having prejudged another human being.

Yet parts of our society are characterised by overt intolerance and discrimination based on others' immigration status and ethnicity. This book challenges any prejudgement of 'foreigners', of migrants and refugees by pointing to the range of motivations that lead to international migration, by outlining that integration differs from assimilation and by stressing the contributions made by migrants.

Empirically the book is based on research conducted among migrant nurses in Britain. However, the principles underpinning these examples equally apply to other professions or migrants in general terms. With increasing globalisation, international migration is here to stay. It affects not just Western, industrialised nations who are often viewed as presenting a 'pull' factor as they can offer a better income and quality of life than those countries migrants originate from. There is also migration within the poorest nations, with people fleeing rural areas in search of better prospects in urban cities. Then there is forced migration due to armed conflicts or natural disasters with the poorest countries hosting the majority of refugees or internally displaced people.

Taking the example of migrant nurses who are either recruited directly to work here or who have migrated independently, often for non-work-related reasons, they make up a large percentage of the shortfall in Britain's nursing labour force. Thus the NHS and independent healthcare sector depend on migrants' contributions in order to meet the required quota of nurses per numbers of patients. At the same time this outflow of nurses leads to a serious brain drain with effects on the delivery of healthcare in many African countries. The number of doctors in Zambia has decreased from 1600 a few years ago to just

400 now, while there are not enough nurses in Botswana to distribute and administer anti-retroviral drugs to people affected by HIV/AIDS.

The stories told by migrant nurses in this book are illustrations of their motivations, their experiences of integrating into the workplace and the contributions they make. Even though they are individual examples, their stories should not be seen in isolation. Each nurse presents a network of contacts and experiences, here as well as in other countries, and these create their individual identities – to be discovered, respected and shared.

Andrea Winkelmann-Gleed
AndreaAWG@aol.com
December 2005

About the author

Dr Andrea Winkelmann-Gleed is a Research Fellow working for the Working Lives Research Institute, based at the London Metropolitan University. Her expertise is in the analysis of international migration, the integration of ethnic minorities and organisational behaviour with a particular focus on the healthcare sector in Britain. In a recent project she has analysed migrant working in the East of England. She holds an Economic and Social Research Council-funded PhD from the School of Development Studies, University of East Anglia, Norwich (2004). She also holds an MSc in Industrial Relations and Personnel Management from the London School of Economics (2000), is a member of the Chartered Institute of Personnel and Development (CIPD) and has a further MSc in International Health from Queen Margaret University College, Edinburgh (1996). For over 14 years she has worked as a project manager in Cambodia, Sudan, Djibouti, Ethiopia and among Rwandan refugees in Tanzania and as researcher and Human Resources manager in England.

Acknowledgements

My appreciation goes out to the hundreds of migrant nurses who have participated in shaping this book by sharing their stories of motivation, integration and contribution to the British healthcare system. The original idea for the research underpinning this book goes back to 2000 when I engaged in discussions with John Eversley from ppre Ltd and Helen Watts from Praxis Community Projects Ltd about the plight of migrant nurses and particularly those who had entered Britain as asylum seekers and had become refugees. Over the following years many people from within and outside the healthcare sector have shared their experiences and perceptions of migration and integration with me and I am grateful to all of them, as they have expanded my own understanding. Alas, I can only mention a few by name. I am grateful for the inputs of my colleagues from the School of Development Studies, namely Janet Seeley and Steve Russell, who have patiently supported me throughout the journey of trying to understand integration; Ben Rogaly from IDS, University of Sussex, who has helped me to disentangle some of the labelling used in describing migrants; Elizabeth Aninonwu from the Mary Seacole Centre for Nursing Practice at Thames Valley University; my colleagues from the Working Lives Research Institute, particularly Sonia McKay and Steve Jefferys, who have given me the space to engage in the adventure of writing this book. Throughout my journey of engaging with migrant nurses, Richard's continuous affection, sense of humour and insight have been crucial to me seeing this project through. Last but not least, my thanks go out to my publishers from Radcliffe Publishing, whose professional support has brought about this end product. If the book brings hope to some migrant nurses and smoothes the path of their integration then it has been a worthwhile mission.

> Administer true justice; show mercy and compassion to one another.
> Do not oppress the foreigner or the poor.
>
> Zechariah 7: 9, 10

CHAPTER 1

Setting the scene

Migration

The example of migrant nurses in Britain stands synonymous for other groups of migrant workers in other Western countries. The analysis of the motivation, integration and contribution of internationally qualified nurses to the health sector presented in this book is based on well established and internationally recognised concepts, making some of the findings accessible and equally transferable to other employment settings.

Migrant nurses are one example of international migration and the steadily increasing numbers of migrants filling jobs that are not filled by indigenous citizens, often for less pay and under worse working conditions; they express a global change in people's mobility. Some of these workers come as seasonal labourers to work on farms and in factories, whereas others are highly skilled Information Technology professionals, researchers or consultants who work as part of multinational companies, symbolising increasing globalisation.

Sentiments towards migrants are split, with highly skilled professionals receiving little criticism and other, less well qualified migrants being viewed as a threat: 'Today, we are being swamped by people arriving illegally from a multitude of countries and cultures, who care nothing for Britain, our traditions or our way of life' wrote Littlejohn in *The Sun* on 9 May 2003. It was suggested that 'immigrants who wish to become British citizens will have to take courses in modern family life and be taught about tolerance of different ethnic groups, unmarried couples and homosexuals'.[1] Hardly a week goes by without some comment in the press on migrants reflecting a dynamic debate surrounding international migration and integration, highlighting a desire to control people flows by distinguishing between the 'wanted' and 'unwanted'. However, such public perceptions, which are not exclusive to Britain, stray far from the facts on worldwide migration and the contribution that migrants are making to the economy and civil society.[2]

Often the terminology surrounding migration, such as 'migrants', 'immigrants', 'asylum seekers' and 'foreigners', is used very lightly, not just by the general public, but also in professional contexts and publications. Recognising that there are overlaps and sometimes blurred boundaries, it is nevertheless paramount to set out some of the definitions at the beginning of this book.

The TUC[3] distinguishes between *migrants*, who came to Britain for the purpose of work; *immigrants*, who came to settle and may become citizens; and *refugees*, who have sought and were granted asylum in Britain on grounds of fear of persecution. While their applications are considered, in Britain by the Home Office, refugees are referred to as *asylum seekers*.

Another distinction is that of *voluntary migration* for economic- or family-related reasons and *forced migration* when asylum seekers are forced to leave their home countries for fear of their safety.

Then there are *undocumented* and *irregular migrants* who may work in the 'grey' economy and move around illegally. They place themselves at great risk and are frequently abused as cheap labourers by being paid less than the National Minimum wage, having deductions for accommodation or transport made from their pay and being subjected to long working days in poor, unregulated working conditions.

The term *migrant workers* is therefore often very loosely defined and there is no one agreed definition; some refer to migrant workers as those who entered the country within the last five years and whose migration is economically motivated. Some migrant workers may only stay for a few months and return again at a later stage, thus becoming *seasonal migrants*. In many countries there are also significant people flows as a result of internal migration, with people moving within international boundaries from one part of a country to another in a search for jobs and economic gain. It also has to be recognised that none of these categories are clear-cut and people can belong to more than one category.

In this book the term *migrant nurse* is used interchangeably with *internationally qualified nurse*, regardless of their motive for migration and regardless of the time of their arrival in the country. It is acknowledged that the term 'internationally qualified' may be less politically laden, but these nurses are clearly participants in today's international migration process. In the case of internationally qualified migrant nurses, the majority are directly recruited through agencies from their countries of origin, often the Philippines, Africa or India, and numbers in Britain have been steadily increasing over the last five years. Yet a second group of internationally qualified nurses migrates independently of agency recruitment and often comes for non-work-related reasons, such as joining their family, getting married, studying for a degree or to seek asylum. As will be outlined in the course of this book, their access to work and integration into the workplace differs from the first group, as they do not enjoy the security of having come to Britain as part of a larger cohort of migrant nurses.

Migration into Britain in context

Until recently migrants were seen as being male with women as dependent spouses.[4,5] In Britain this led the Immigration Appellate Authority to develop Asylum Gender Guidelines,[6] intended to ensure that the gender of asylum seekers does not prejudice their application.

Within the British context, migration has to be viewed within a wider perspective of her unique historical links to other countries and her imperial past, with waves of migrants and immigrants from Asia, Africa and the West Indies.[7] Historically, after the Suez crisis in 1956, Britain had to come to terms with a postcolonial world,[8] as a result of which Britain's migrant labour experience was partially characterised by Commonwealth citizens setting up their home in Britain as they had, until 1967, a right to live here. Therefore Britain's migrant labour experience differs from the rest of Western Europe since Commonwealth citizens, as a result of their legal status, were more privileged than, for example, Turks and Greeks who immigrated to Germany as 'guestworkers'. During the 1950s and 1960s Commonwealth citizens contributed to Britain's economy by filling socially undesirable jobs and the rebuilding of war-shattered Britain created a demand for labour that was met through immigration from the Indian subcontinent and the Caribbean. This demand for workers was also particularly acute in the National Health Service (NHS), with Indian doctors being actively recruited in the 1950s[9] and large numbers of nurses coming from the Caribbean in the 1950s and 1960s – a phenomenon that continues to this day. Yet the effects of immigration and integration into Britain have been, and are currently probably more than ever, the subject of fierce debate.[10]

Despite this seeming generosity towards immigrants, Crewe *et al.* point out that many people from formerly colonised countries who came to Britain in the hope of finding a modern, civilised and progressive place to live were disappointed with the working conditions they found.[11] Despite the demand for labour, Black and Asian workers were treated as 'second-class' employees, with open discrimination being common practice in management approaches during the post-World War II period. Even though immigration to Britain was partially triggered by labour shortage, the economic upheaval of the 1970s led to the perception that 'they' came here to take 'our' jobs, an attitude that persists to this day.[12,13] Britain's history of colonial domination and migration affects people's attitudes towards migrants and the migrants' subsequent integration at their place of employment, as the example of Asian and Afro-Caribbean workers shows.[14]

However, the question remains to what extent these nurses have truly integrated and to what extent they were encouraged to develop their careers. It is reported that the typical Health Care Assistant, providing a backbone to the NHS yet being relatively unqualified, is 40–50 years old and of Asian or

Afro-Caribbean origin. This implies that many nurses who migrated to Britain are filling vacancies and are stuck in low-skilled, low-paid grades. So, to what extent have integration strategies, equal opportunities policies and diversity management techniques really had an impact on the role and perception of migrant nurses? How have things changed from Mary Seacole's days?

> Mary Seacole was born in Jamaica, where she learned nursing skills from her mother, who kept a boarding house for invalid soldiers. Mary came to Britain in 1845, where she applied to the War Office to offer her services as a nurse to British troops engaged in the Crimean War. However, she was turned down because of colour prejudice. Mary was not discouraged by this and funded her own trip to the Crimea, where she set to nursing the sick and wounded. She also started her own shop, selling medicines. Mary became a favourite with soldiers, one of whom wrote in his memoirs, 'she was a wonderful woman'. After the war, Mary returned to Britain in poor health, but her predicament was brought to public attention by a letter to *The Times*. A benefit was held for her in the Royal Surrey Gardens, which lasted for four days, and Mary was able to live well thereafter. Mary died on 14 May 1881, in London.[15]

As part of the wider business case for immigration, the economic argument that younger migrant workers can contribute to redress the 'pensions' gap has been developed. The report published by Lord Taverne QC[17] estimates that by 2050 48.5% of the British population will be 65 years or older. Furthermore, the UK Home Office admits that in 1999/2000 migrants have made a net fiscal contribution of about £2.5 billion to the economy, thereby contributing more in taxes than they have received in benefits and state services.

Currently, as a result of international migration a substantial number of healthcare workers are non-UK qualified or were not born in the UK: 31% of doctors and 13% of nurses in the NHS are now non-UK born.[16] Some of these came in the 1960s and 70s and had or have later gained British citizenship. In addition there are also around 30 000 non-British nurses working in the NHS, who have no citizenship rights and rely on work permits.

While much of what is said in this book equally applies to employees and nurses in general or Black and minority ethnic nurses specifically, it uses the examples of migrant nurses who have crossed internationally recognised borders to get to Britain, with refugee nurses being one sub-group of international migrants. The next section provides an introduction to the particular situation of refugees.

The worlds' refugees

Britain has historically also offered sanctuary to people groups in crisis: since the late eighteenth century the refugees fleeing to Britain have included Jews,

Ugandan Asians, Vietnamese, Zairians and recently Yugoslavs.[18] Yet Britain's response to refugees has seen a changing perception of asylum seekers over the past 15 years. Until the early 1980s they were seen as brave people, fleeing persecution. In the mid-1980s it was with the arrival of young Tamil men from Sri Lanka seeking asylum from persecution that a perception that refugees might be 'bogus' developed. Unlike in other European countries, the Tamils were hardly ever given asylum in Britain.[19] Single young men from South Asia were the people against whom UK immigration control was targeted, as there was a culture of disbelief that they were 'genuine' refugees. Such attitudes were informed by a lack of understanding of economic and political instabilities as a result of endemic ethnic persecution. Kurdish, Somali, Kosovan and Albanian asylum seekers were subsequently classified as 'bogus' and deterred from coming to Britain.

Within the international scope of forced migration, figures of asylum seekers in Europe and indeed in Britain are comparatively insignificant: international refugee data show the highest numbers of displaced persons come from the Middle East[20] and in 2001 over three million people were forcibly displaced within Africa. For example, Tanzania hosted half a million refugees from the Great Lakes region and Sudan 370 000. In comparison, based on ICRC reports in 2001 the whole of Europe only hosted 960 500 refugees, with nearly half of these displaced from Yugoslavia. Out of these Britain had received 67 700 applications for asylum and Germany nearly twice that number. The ICRC figures on refugee migration correspond with those published by UNHCR[21] and those published by the UK Home Office.[22] In 2005 Refugees International estimates the number of displaced in Darfur to be 700 000 and out of these approximately 180 000 have crossed the international border into neighbouring Chad.[23] Thus with most people fleeing to neighbouring countries, some of the poorest countries are hosting the bulk of refugees.

However, there has been a rise in the number of asylum applications to Britain since the 1990s,[24] indicative of the rising numbers of independent migrants. In 2000 the total number of asylum seekers in Britain rose to 80 315 and in 2002 to over 100 000, with the main applicant nationalities coming from the Federal Republic of Yugoslavia, Iraq, Iran, Sri Lanka and Afghanistan. Over recent years the number of asylum-related grants of settlement has been going down.

The Control of Immigration Statistics for 2003 show a 30% decrease compared to the previous year.[25] In 2003 the Home Office received 46 130 asylum appeals, 11% fewer than in 2002 and one in five (20%) appeals were granted, compared with 22% in 2002.

On the 22 February 2005 BBC News reported the following update on the UK's asylum figures: some 34 000 people sought asylum in the UK in 2004 compared with 49 000 in 2003. Figures for the first quarter of 2005 show that the number of applicants, excluding dependants, fell by 17% compared to the previous three months. In 2005, the top three nationalities seeking asylum were Iranian, Iraqi and Somali people. Of the cases considered during the quarter, some 6% were granted asylum and a further 10% were allowed humanitarian protection or discretionary leave, with 84% being refused.[26] Separate figures from the UN's refugee agency are expected to show that this is in line with continued falls in asylum arrivals across Europe.

The Home Office and refugee organisations estimate that over half of the international migrants coming to the UK settle in London.[27] The total number of refugees who have entered Britain over the last 15 years and are now living in London is estimated to be between 240 000 and 280 000, but there are no reliable, published sources for this.[28,29] Efforts to stem people flows into Britain and to address what is commonly called the 'asylum and immigration crisis' have culminated in the White Paper *Secure Borders, Safe Haven*,[30] which led to the 2002 Nationality, Immigration and Asylum Bill.[31] Asylum seekers might possess professional skills, which are sought after in Britain, yet these are not taken into consideration when processing their claims.[32] With Europe tightening immigration controls and visa constraints, it has become virtually impossible for someone fleeing for safety to reach Britain legally even though they might comply with the 1951 Geneva Convention.[33] The involvement of paid middle-men is therefore common practice, which can lead to further endangerment and abuse of individuals who are already vulnerable.

The Home Office sets out aims of what an integration strategy of asylum seekers and refugees into British society should achieve, namely:

- to include refugees as equal members of society
- to help refugees develop their potential and contribute to the cultural and economic life of the country
- to set out a clear framework to support the integration process across the UK
- to facilitate access to the support necessary for the integration of refugees nationally and regionally.

However, despite providing a policy of immigration, the government fails to provide a clearer definition of what is understood by 'integration'. In relation to refugees the Home Office describes integration as follows:

> Recognised refugees are entitled to the same social and economic rights as UK citizens and have full access to medical treatment, education, housing and employment. Recognised refugees have an obligation to conform to the laws of their country of refuge.[34]

With a lack of definition of the deeper meaning of 'integration', this statement refers to the refugees' access to basic services and their responsibility to obey the rules of the land. The government further acknowledges that employment is a key factor in their integration.[35] Some research has been undertaken to look at the skills that migrants in general may have to offer and the barriers they face when trying to integrate into employment,[36–9] and the National Refugee Integration Forum looks at all aspects of how refugees integrate into British society.

Eastmond draws on the example of Chilean refugees in the United States of America and points out that female migrants experienced greater self-reliance and confidence as a result of employment. In comparison the men felt that with the loss of social and political networks work had lost some of its deeper meaning.[40] Eastmond describes how these men find themselves in a paradox with 'the torment of remembering and the fear of forgetting'. This shows that migration and employment has an immense impact on personal and work-related identities as individuals lose their familiar points of reference and need to establish new ones as part of the integration process. Migration leads to changes in childcare arrangements, kinship and community support and gaining access to employment can affect men and women in different ways, depending on their skills and culture of origin.

Against the backdrop of the current policy debates and historic cases of migration, this book questions the validity of the one-sided public opinions about migrants and integration by scrutinising personal perspectives of living and working in another country. It looks at how facets of individual- and work-related identities, their interface with motivation and the management of diversity act as contributors for migrants to make a positive contribution.

References

1   Woolf M (2002) Immigrants who seek British citizenship will have to take lessons in tolerance. *The Independent*. **29 October**: 1.

2   Gott G and Johnson K (2002) *The Migrant Population in the UK: fiscal effects*. Home Office, London.

3   TUC (2002) *Migrant Workers: a TUC guide*. TUC and JCWI, London.

4   Harzig C (2003) Immigration policies: a gendered historical comparison. In: M Morokvasic-Müller, U Erel and K Shinozaki (eds) *Crossing Borders and Shifting Boundaries*. Vol 1: Gender on the Move. Leske and Budrich, Opladen, Germany.

5   Knocke W (2000) Migrant and ethnic minority women: the effects of gender neutral legislation in the European Union. In: B Hobson (ed) *Gender and Citizenship in Transition*. Routledge, London.

6   IAA (2000) *Asylum Gender Guidelines*. Immigration Appellate Authority, London.

7   Panayi P (1999) *The Impact of Immigration: a documentary history of the effects and experiences of immigrants in Britain since 1945*. Manchester University Press, Manchester.

8   Ramdin R (1999) *Reimaging Britain: 500 years of Black and Asian history*. Pluto Press, London.

9   Coker N (2001) *Racism in Medicine: an agenda for change.* King's Fund Publishing, London.

10   Modood T, Berthoud R, Lakey J *et al.* (1997) *Ethnic Minorities in Britain: diversity and disadvantage.* Policy Studies Institute, London.

11   Crewe E and Kothari U (1998) Gujurati migrants search for modernity in Britain. *Gender and Development.* **6**(1): 13–20.

12   Banks M (1996) *Ethnicity: anthropological constructions.* Routledge, London.

13   Kessler S and Bayliss F (1998) *Contemporary British Industrial Relations* (3e). Macmillan Business, London.

14   Baxter C (2001) *Managing Diversity and Inequality in Health Care.* Harcourt Publishers Limited, London.

15   Mary Seacole. www.mckenziehpa.com/bw/tenview.html#seacole.

16   Findlay A (2002) *From Brain Exchange to Brain Gain: policy implications for the UK of recent trends in skilled migration from developing countries.* International Labour Office, International Migration Branch, Geneva.

17   Lord Taverne QC, Benedetti D, Bolkenstein CF *et al.* (2001) *Pension Compendium: pensions reform in Europe.* The Federal Trust for Education and Research, London.

18   Bunting M (2001) Haven't we been here before? Welcome to Britain. *The Guardian.* **23 May:** 92–4.

19   Parekh B (2000) *The Future of Multi-ethnic Britain: the Parekh Report.* The Runnymede Trust, London.

20   International Committee of the Red Cross (2002) *World Disasters Report 2002: focus on reducing risk.* International Federation of the Red Cross and Red Crescent Societies, Geneva.

21   United Nations High Commissioner for Refugees (2002) *Trends in Asylum Applications Lodged in Europe, North America, Australia and New Zealand, 2001.* UNHCR, Geneva.

22   Home Office (2002) *Asylum Statistics 2002. United Kingdom.* Home Office, London. www.ncadc.org.uk/letters/newszine32/stats2002.html.

23   Refugees International (2004) Sudan: continuing displacement and incalculable death in Darfur. www.refugeesinternational.org/content/article/detail/938?PHPSESSID= 6e98e287ab6ee04598a437226c27e48a.

24   Home Office (2001) *Asylum Statistics: April 2001 United Kingdom.* Home Office, London. www.homeoffice.gov.uk/rds/pdfs2/hosb902.pdf.

25   Dudley (2004) *Control of Immigration: Statistics. UK 2003. Home Office Statistical Bulletin.* Home Office, London.

26   Home Office (2005) *Asylum Statistics First Quarter.* The Home Office, London. www. homeoffice.gov.uk/rds/pdfs05/asylumq105.pdf.

27   London Research Centre (2002) *The Capital Divided: asylum statistics. United Kingdom 1997.* London Research Centre, London. www.londonshealth.gov.uk/pdf/lhs/ hsfact2.pdf.

28 Lewis R (1997) The Demographics and Geographics of London's Ethnic Minorities. London Research Centre, London.

29 Cairncross F (2002) *The Longest Journey: a survey of migration*. The Economist, London.

30 Home Office (2002) *Secure Borders, Safe Haven: integration with diversity in modern Britain*. White Paper. The Stationery Office, London.

31 Home Office (2002) *Nationality, Immigration and Asylum Bill*. Home Office, London.

32 Refugee Council (2002) *Government Announcement and Proposals Since its White Paper on Asylum: a summary*. The Refugee Council, London.

33 Burnett A and Peel M (2001) The health of survivors of torture and organised violence, asylum seekers and refugees in Britain. *BMJ*. **322**: 606–9.

34 Home Office (2003) Refugee integration, Vol. 2003: IND (Immigration Nationality Directorate). http://www.ind.homeoffice.gov.uk/ind/en/home/laws_policy/refugee_integration0.html

35 DWP (Department for Work and Pensions) (2003) *Working to Rebuild Lives: a preliminary report towards a refugee employment strategy. Draft report*. Disadvantaged Groups Division, Department for Work and Pensions, Sheffield.

36 Bloch A (2002) Refugees' opportunities and barriers in employment and training. Department of Works and Pensions, Leeds.

37 Cabinet Office (1999) *Equal Opportunities Monitoring Guidance, Version 2*. Cabinet Office, Corporate Strategy and Diversity Division, London.

38 Cabinet Office (2003) *Ethnic Minorities and the Labour Market*. Cabinet Office, Strategy Unit, London.

39 Dumper H (2002) Missed opportunities, a skills audit of refugee women in London from the teaching, nursing and medical professions. Mayor of London in Association with Refugee Women's Association, London.

40 Eastmond M (1993) Reconstructing lives: Chilean refugee women. In: G Buijs (ed) *Migrant Women: crossing boundaries and changing identities*. Berg, Oxford.

CHAPTER 2

Identities and boundaries

Race and ethnicity

The debate on migration, immigration and attitudes towards migrants and asylum seekers is closely linked to the interpretation of race and ethnicity informing relationships and identities. The concepts of race, migration and ethnicity are indistinct and writing on migrant minority ethnic groups in Britain has focused on Blacks and Asians, with the term 'Black' referring to those who can trace their ancestors to the Caribbean and former colonies in Africa, especially Nigeria and Ghana, and the term 'Asian' referring to people from South Asia, primarily India, Pakistan and Bangladesh, but not China.[1] As with migration, race relations need to be seen within the context of the nation.[2]

The terms 'ethnic', 'ethnicity' and 'race' are often being used interchangeably, contributing further to the heated and muddled debate on immigration and integration. As a result, even though there are numerous definitions, these overlap and fail to be concise. Epstein argues that the individual's perception of identity is influenced by external, social factors as well as internal psychological ones.[3] Thus ethnic identity develops as a lifelong process. Yet the term 'ethnic identity' is elusive, as it is based on self-perception as well as the perception of others.[4] It implies identification with people one views as similar to oneself, referring to features of culture, religion and language, yet these are subjective and do not necessarily correspond among groups, as the ethnic conflicts in the Balkan region show. Neither do ethnic groups correspond with nations, which are often multi-ethnic.[5]

The term 'race' is usually defined by physical characteristics, such as skin pigmentation or the shape of eyes and nose. It is laden with the historical legacy of a division of the population into different types and the idea that characteristic appearances constitute biological differences.[6] Yet it is part of common thinking and the ordering of social relations. Parekh argues that the term 'race' is now widely acknowledged as a social and political construct and not a biological, genetic one, thus applying it interchangeably with ethnicity. Hence to define 'ethnic groups' as complex social constructs and 'race' as a biological, quasi-scientific phenomenon would be misleading.[7] For example, 'ethnic monitoring', conducted by many employers as part of their implementation of equal opportunities policies, relies on 'racial' characteristics or geographical boundaries, such as 'Black African' or 'Mixed – White and Asian'. Such classifications do not give the respondent any opportunity to express their deeper ethnic identity, which includes values and beliefs. Much of the statistical data on ethnicity or race are therefore used to label individuals in order to manage them in the social system,[8] thus confirming that they are used for political and economic interest.[9]

The term 'prejudice' means 'prejudgement' and refers to an unfavourable attitude towards a social group and its members, with 'racism' being prejudice against people based on their ethnicity or race. Ideologies have been developed in order to mark the 'rulers and ruled' and the 'privileged and underprivileged', with White elites justifying their dominant position.[10] This leads to racism based on genetically transmitted traits or on cultural elements. The discourse of race thinking, resulting in racism, was developed within a context of political domination and economic exploitation.[11,12] Genocide is the ultimate expression of this attitude.[13] A mindset of prejudice can lead to discriminatory behaviour towards others, who subsequently feel excluded. This process can take place anywhere in public life, including work.

Yet it is more difficult to alter practice than to issue policy documents. According to Gill, although 30% of all doctors in the UK are from 'ethnic minorities' and it is estimated that there are 2000 'refugee doctors' in the country,[14] nevertheless, when competing with a White applicant with similar qualifications for a post, an Asian or Black doctor is likely to be rejected. Indeed some studies on diversity in the NHS go as far as accusing the wider organisational set-up of institutional racism.[15–17] Institutional racism constitutes an established organisation especially of public character displaying *behaviour of prejudice and discrimination*. It resides in the policies, procedures, operations and culture of institutions and reinforces prejudices and in turn is reinforced by them. In cases of institutional racism the individual can suffer silently under discrimination and harassment for many years and it can be very difficult to identify and change once certain practices have become integral features of organisational culture. More apparent is the under-representation of people from ethnic minorities in NHS management roles, which causes concern among advocates for equality.[18–19]

Moreover, historic events formed terms such as 'ethnic cleansing', 'ethnic hatred', 'genocide' and 'anti-Semitism'. These prejudices are directed at a group of people who may share beliefs or language, a geographical region or racial characteristics in any combination or be perceived by others in this way. Thus a definition of 'racism' which includes *any form of discrimination on the basis of race or ethnicity* is adopted in this book. Such racial stereotyping shows that the perceptions of 'others' – here those showing hostility towards a 'stranger', someone who is 'different' – differ from that of the 'self', who is made up of multiple identities and not just racial or ethnic ones.

For example, a Black or Asian person can be British and may have lived here all their lives, yet some White British citizens may only notice physical characteristics and conclude 'strangeness' rather than familiarity of shared nationhood.[20] Consequently such individuals perceived as 'strangers' may be linked to crime, to infections such as AIDS, to low skill levels and ultimately to 'them' and 'us' thinking. This perception that physical characteristics, such as skin pigmentation, play an important part in power relations, which affect the way the White 'host' country relates to minority groups, is a point that seems to have been missed by some anthropologists according to Banks.

There can be a sense of identity and belonging between members of certain minority ethnic groups, particularly when they share a common language or religious tradition.[21,22] For example this becomes visible in the way nurses from certain African or Afro-Caribbean countries bond with each other.[23,24] Therefore even if these groups of nurses face racial discrimination from a dominant 'other', they receive support from each other and the shared experience of hostility, relating to the concept of in- and out-groups. When such socialisation takes place, successful workplace integration may not be the result of good management and high levels of job satisfaction, but that of collectively facing a perceived threat. As Tajfel[25] and Morris[26] point out, members of minority groups can feel some commonality in race, nationality, culture and history and in addition may share experiences of discrimination and social disadvantage in their host community.

Taken to the extreme, this attitude may even partially explain why so many migrant nurses who entered Britain in the 1950s and 60s have not significantly progressed in their careers. Being a minority, they may have adopted a defeatist attitude and reinforced this among each other. While such a conclusion is highly provocative, it should be noted that only a few studies have looked at nurses' workplace integration and all have noted significant levels of discrimination and even institutional racism.[27,28] In the early years of people migrating to Britain it appeared obvious that they were 'only' filling vacancies and their integration into the workforce and right to be treated equally and fairly was not asserted by them or their employers. Therefore, as Modood *et al.*[29] point out, discrimination against manual and public sector workers was integral in industrial relations during the post-World War II years. Consequently group cohesion can be one of a number of factors affecting integration and workplace behaviour.

Equality and integration

As part of the wider integration process in a host country, employment becomes a key expression, providing migrants with dignity, confidence and economic as well as emotional stability.[30,31] Ahmed argues that employment can enhance the feeling of belonging within a foreign place.[32] By going out to work like most other people, points of identity with them can arise. The 'stranger' becomes a familiar feature for 'natives' and differences can be overlaid through the discovery of similarities. Thus the stranger does not have to assimilate, but, at best, the focus can turn from facets of distinction to acceptance and an integration of diversity. At worst, the recognition of difference can lead to exclusion and expressions of unfairness and intolerance by the majority as the stranger may be perceived as a threat and accused of taking 'our' jobs. This interaction with others, colleagues and supervisors in particular, gives work further meaning provided it is managed properly.

Recently there has been a growing interest in the management of diversity within the British healthcare sector, reflected in a range of publications.[33–6] It has to be acknowledged that the terminology of diversity is less explicit than that related to equal opportunities, which seeks to address racism and discrimination.

Some groups of Black and minority ethnic nurses migrated to Britain from the Caribbean and Africa in the 1950s and 60s while others have only recently been recruited from overseas. Yet organisational- and behavioural studies have considered nurses as one homogenous group of people and have reported on their job satisfaction[37] and their management in hospitals.[38–40]

Diversity is referred to on an individual, but also on wider levels. Hofstede[41] with his publication of *Culture's Consequences* and Trompenaars *et al.*[42] have clarified differences in national culture through differences in behaviours in organisations. This kind of research has been conducted in multinational business corporations and carries the danger of oversimplifying national cultures. However, the relationships between facets of migrants' identities and aspects of their working lives have so far only received little attention.[43]

Many Black and minority ethnic people are socially excluded in Britain with social exclusion referring to a process brought about by lack of economic, political and social citizenship leading to a lack of access to financial services, participation in decision making, social networks, relations and helpful contacts.[44]

> Social exclusion is a phenomenon of alienation and distance from society . . .
> Exclusion is the fact of preventing, even temporarily, someone from participating in social relationships and the construction of society.[45]

Social exclusion can be caused by a range of factors and Narayan *et al.*[46] have, for example, identified poverty, lack of money and power; ethnic, racial, linguistic and cultural isolation; ill health and disabilities; behaviours that are outside the norm; exclusion of women and self-exclusion. Sen draws attention to the distinction between active and passive exclusion, with 'active exclusion' describing the situation of refugees and immigrants who suffer deprivations as a result of not being given political status.[47] 'Passive exclusion' refers to deprivation as a result of social processes, for example economic problems leading to poverty and isolation.

Such exclusion can be closely linked to the lack of integration of 'the stranger' who is different and does not belong, a concept outlined by Ahmed.[32] The stranger is recognised as 'not belonging' as a result of being 'different' to the norm. This can encompass differences related to gender, migration and ethnicity. These notions of cultural 'otherness' and 'difference' help to sustain the boundaries between White British and Black and minority ethnic individuals.

Yet migration and being 'a migrant' is more complex than just being a stranger. It encompasses identity, belonging and home in relation to a particular space, history, movement and dislocation. Thus it pays attention to visible and invisible differences, also labelled as deep- and surface-level diversity.[48,49] Surface-level diversity reflected in the blurred boundaries and muddled understandings of race, ethnicity and migration leads to prejudices among people who are 'different'.

Social exclusion and the integration of people from different cultural backgrounds into public life have now become part of the British political agenda. The Race Relations Act (1976) makes:

> Discrimination unlawful on the grounds of colour, race, nationality or ethnic or national origin in employment and other fields. It is unlawful to discriminate against a person either directly or indirectly on these grounds.

The British Race Relations Act 1976 led to the establishment of the Commission for Racial Equality (CRE), whose duties are to eliminate racial discrimination, promote equality and monitor the implementation of the Act.[50] The CRE and Equal Opportunities Commission have issued Codes of Practice for employers, aiming to eliminate discrimination in employment, which are not legally binding, but admissible as evidence in industrial tribunals.[51] As a result of the Stephen Lawrence Inquiry, the Race Relations Amendment Act was passed and as of April 2000 it imposes an obligation on public, including the NHS, bodies to have a Race Equality Scheme consisting of targets to reduce incidences of harassment at work and actively promote equality.[52] Now managers are held responsible for racial equality in their organisations.[53] Higher than average levels of unemployment among minority ethnic groups in Britain and their under-representation in management roles indicate that the reality differs from what the law sets out to achieve. Recently some policymakers have acknowledged underlying prejudices in the British healthcare sector. Commonly the literature on 'ethnic minorities in Britain' does not distinguish between immigrants who can be 'second generation immigrants' and refugees. Even though issues related to HR management and discrimination equally apply to both groups, refugees are even more disadvantaged. Often they face extreme financial hardship, have suffered psychological distress and are ambiguous about their legal status and future. These studies signify that people of minority ethnic identity are still socially constructed as 'other', rather than as 'normal'.

Migration, ethnicity and gender related to employment

Existing figures only show that higher than average numbers of non-White workers are in less desirable jobs. Recent census data show a rise in the already very high unemployment rate for Black and minority ethnic groups, particularly for Pakistanis and Bangladeshis, even though it has decreased for Whites between 1991 and 2001, as the following table shows:

Table 2.1   Unemployment by ethnic group in Britain

Ethnicity	Unemployment rate 1991	Unemployment rate 2001
White	6%	4.7%
Indian	8%	7.3%
Black (all in 1991/other in 2001)	19%	16.4%
Black African	–	14.1%
Black Caribbean	–	11.6%
Bangladeshi and Pakistani	21%	37.4%
Chinese	–	6.0%
Mixed	–	12.4%

Source: Khan (1991) and 2001 Census.[54]

It is hardly possible to find any reliable statistics on the numbers and professional backgrounds of migrants or refugees who are working in the UK. In relation to refugee nurses, Eversley *et al.*[55] have identified barriers that prevent their access to employment and subsequent integration. In relation to migrant workers one conclusion was that many work below their skill levels in low-skilled, low-paid jobs.[56] The lack of procedures to recognise professional qualification and the lack of suitable conversion courses or work placements add to the fact that many migrants are unable to fulfil their true potential. Added to that are the hurdles related to language skills and personal issues related to childcare, financial constraints, housing, immigration status, lack of documents to prove past training and experience as well as cultural and psychological issues. In some cases added barriers of discrimination, experience of torture and domestic violence can play a role too.

Since 31 May 2002 the race equality duty requires public authorities to monitor their functions and policies for any adverse impact on race equality and to assess the likely impact of any proposed policies on the promotion of race equality.[57] This means that they have to adopt ethnic monitoring systems which to date are not consistently implemented. Therefore it is difficult to give an accurate breakdown of the ethnicity of Britain's nursing staff.

Existing studies on migrant nurses suggest that they are under-represented in senior grades, denied career progression and kept in auxiliary positions and less desirable clinical specialities.[58] Moreover, there are reports of extensive discrimination on a personal and institutional level leading to wide-ranging racial inequality, thus making the experiences of internationally qualified nurses symbolic of migrants in a range of professions.

It also remains a global struggle to attract men into nursing and it is, therefore, unremarkable that the growing number of publications on migrant nurses assumes them to be female, confirming that nursing generally is viewed as a woman's occupation.[59-64] When a nurse is a man, a qualifier is often used: he is a 'male nurse'.[65] de Lange[66] goes further by suggesting that the usual categorisation is that 'nurses are single whereas doctors have wives' because they are male.

Evans[67] describes how prevailing definitions of masculinity act as a barrier to men's entry to nursing in Canada, Britain and the United States. This view is supported by a Swedish study from Öhlén et al.,[68] who report that members of the public voiced their uncertainty over interacting with a male rather than with a female nurse. However, not only the public may resent the presence of a male nurse. In a British study on the gendered interaction between doctors and nurses, a male nurse commented that he felt threatened and disempowered by the gender discourse and his female colleagues' perception of a 'real' nurse.[69] It is ironic that stereotypical notions of masculinity seem to pressure men into some of the best-paying and most prestigious nursing specialities.[70] MacDougall[71] explains that while men often enter nursing for the same reasons as women – a desire to care for others, perceived job security and the power that accrues to a professional position – the pressure (from themselves or others) to conform to stereotypes of the 'dominant male' causes many to move away from caring roles into managerial positions.

Gender divisions are often based on a patriarchal model of gender roles, which ascribes 'caring' attributes to women and 'rational', 'instrumental', 'managerial' attributes to men.[72-76] McNay[77] states that gender identity is not just a result of patriarchal structures, but also of a set of norms that are reflected in the customary practices of men and women. Almost universally women are portrayed by men and themselves as 'dependants' or 'victims' of male violence, oppression, economic development and religion.[78-79] This is for example compounded by viewing a housewife merely as holding a 'maintenance function', compared to the 'productive role', which is held by male wage earners.

Women constitute three-quarters of the NHS workforce in Britain and just under 90% of nurses are female. While nursing continues to be an 'overwhelmingly female profession', the number of registered male nurses has been very gradually increasing: 9.89% in 2001, 10.21% in 2002 and 10.48% in 2003.[80] It is interesting to note, given the low numbers of male nurses registered in Britain, that out of the 220 nurses on a database for refugee nurses held by the Royal College of Nursing and Midwifery 29.4% are male.[81] Many of the male nurses choose specialties like psychiatric nursing, casualty or intensive care.[82] In the NHS it is women who are concentrated in lower-paid jobs, such as cleaning, catering, nursing, paramedical, ancillary and clerical positions,[83] yet women are under-represented in management positions. Despite attempts to challenge this, looking after sick people continues to be seen as an extension of tasks viewed as 'feminine' and the presence of male nurses still confronts common perceptions of masculinity.

Therefore some inter-occupational inequalities in healthcare employment are linked to gender, with a male managerial elite and nurses looking after sick people seen as an extension of tasks viewed as 'feminine'; the presence of male nurses can challenge common perceptions of masculinity. Each culture has its own gender system and aspects of this carry on in the process of migration to Britain and influence integration.[84,85] Data from the Labour Force Survey[86] confirm that gender, migration and ethnicity have a negative impact on women's employment: first, fewer women are in managerial roles than men and second, there are even fewer women from Black and minority ethnic backgrounds in managerial responsibility with negligible figures for Bangladeshi/ Pakistani women.

In addition, the immigration and asylum law is written from a framework of male experiences, viewing them as the breadwinner.[87,88] This leads to the assumption that gender roles have a role to play in the process of migration and subsequent integration and employment which affects masculinities and femininities. Moreover, in employment women may find themselves being treated as racially as well as sexually inferior.[89]

Ely concluded that an organisation's demographic structure, which includes 'gender', plays an important role in the identification process of its members.[90] Williams *et al.* elaborated on this by stating that women construct their identity by drawing comparisons between themselves and men.[91] Hence even though women and men may integrate differently, women are more vulnerable to abuse and may find access to employment more difficult or may choose not to work for cultural reasons. Moreover much of their work is related to an extension of their 'mothering and care-taking' roles.[92,93] Thus ethnicity and gender seem to impact on whether someone gains employment and subsequently benefits from the effects that this may have on wider integration.[94] In this book aspects of gender are examined in relation to migration, ethnicity and employment.

References

1   Banks M (1996) *Ethnicity: anthropological constructions*. Routledge, London.

2   Banton M (1983) *Racial and Ethnic Competition*. Cambridge University Press, Cambridge.

3   Epstein AL (1978) *Ethos and Identity: three studies in ethnicity*. Tavistock, London.

4   Hutnik N (1991) *Ethnic Minority Identity: a social psychological perspective*. Oxford University Press, Oxford.

5   Bealey F (1999) *The Blackwell Dictionary of Political Science*. Blackwell Publishers, Oxford.

6   Fenton S (1999) *Ethnicity, Racism, Class and Culture*. Macmillan Press Ltd, London.

7   Parekh B (2000) *Rethinking Multiculturalism: cultural diversity and political theory*. Macmillan Press, London.

8   Morris L (2002) *Managing Migration: civic stratification and migrants' rights*. Routledge, London.

9   Cohen A (1969) *Custom and Politics in Urban Africa: a study of Hausa migrants in Yoruba towns*. Routledge and Kegan Paul, London.

10 Gellner E (1983) *Nations and Nationalism*. Blackwell, Oxford.

11 Wolf E (1982) *Europe and the People Without History*. University of California Press, Berkeley.

12 Stannard DE (1992) *American Holocaust: the conquest of the New World*. Oxford University Press, Oxford.

13 Hogg MA and Vaughan GM (2002) *Social Psychology* (3e). Prentice Hall, London.

14 Gill PS (2001) General Practitioners, ethnic diversity and racism. In: N Coker (2001) *Racism in Medicine: an agenda for change*. King's Fund Publishing, London.

15 Dhruev N (2001) *Racism and Oppression in the NHS: seizing the Macpherson opportunity*. Somerset Partnership NHS Trust.

16 James J and Baxter C (2001) The multiracial team: the challenges ahead. In: C Baxter (ed) *Managing Diversity and Inequality in Health Care*. Baillière Tindall and RCN, London.

17 Coker N (2001) *Racism in Medicine, an agenda for change*. King's Fund Publishing, London.

18 Mwasandube P (2001) Resistance movement. *Nursing Times*. **97**(27): 12–13.

19 Harrison S (2003) White nurses dominate shortlists for senior ranks. *Nursing Standard*. **19 February**. www.nursing-standard.co.uk/thisweek/news3.htm.

20 Hutnik N (1991) *Ethnic Minority Identity: a social psychological perspective*. Oxford University Press, Oxford.

21 Bhopal R (1995) *Ethnicity, Race, Health and Research: racist black box or enlightened epidemiology*. Paper presented at the Society for Social Medicine Scientific Meeting.

22 Collier MJ and Thomas M (1988) Cultural identity: and interpretative perspective. In: YY Kim and WB Gudykunst WB (eds.) *Theories in Intercultural Communication*. Sage, Newbury Park, CA.

23 Beishon S, Virdee S and Hagell A (1995) *Nursing in a Multi-ethnic NHS*. Policy Studies Institute, London.

24 Culley L and Mayor V (2001) Ethnicity and nursing careers. In: L Culley and S Dyson (ed) *Ethnicity and Nursing Practice*. Palgrave, Basingstoke.

25 Tajfel H (1978) *The Social Psychology of Minorities*. Minority Rights Group, London.

26 Morris HS (1968) Ethnic groups. *International Encyclopedia of the Social Sciences*. **2**: 167–72.

27 Culley L and Dyson S (2001) *Ethnicity and Nursing Practice*. Palgrave, Basingstoke.

28 Baxter C (2001) *Managing Diversity and Inequality in Health Care*. Harcourt Publishers Limited, London.

29 Modood T, Berthoud R, Lakey J *et al.* (1997) *Ethnic Minorities in Britain, Diversity and Disadvantage*. Policy Studies Institute, London.

30 Warr P (2002) The study of well-being, behaviour and attitudes. In: P Warr (ed) *Psychology at Work*. Penguin Books, London.

31 Teichmann I (2002) *Credit to the Nation: refugee contributions to the UK*. The Refugee Council, London.

32 Ahmed S (2000) *Strange Encounters: embodied others in post-coloniality*. Routledge, London.

33 Beishon S, Virdee S and Hagell A (1995) *Nursing in a Multi-ethnic NHS*. Policy Studies Institute, London.

34 Holland K and Hogg C (2001) *Cultural Awareness in Nursing and Health Care*. Arnold, London.

35 RCN (2001) *Welcome to the UK, welcome to the RCN*. Royal College of Nursing, London.

36 RCN (2002) *Diversity Appraisal Resource Guide: helping employers, RCN officers and representatives promote diversity in the workplace*. Royal College of Nursing, London.

37 Tovey EJ and Adams AE (1999) The changing nature of nurses' job satisfaction: an exploration of sources of satisfaction in the 1990s. *Journal of Advanced Nursing*. **30**(1): 150–8.

38 Adams A, Bond S and Arber S (1995) Development and validation of scales to measure organisational features of acute hospital wards. *International Journal of Nursing Studies*. **32**(6): 612–27.

39 McNeese-Smith DK (1999) The relationship between managerial motivation, leadership, nurse outcomes and patient satisfaction. *Journal of Organisational Behaviour*. **20**: 243–59.

40 Hofstede G (1981) Management control of public and non-for-profit activities. *Accounting, Organizations and Society*. **6**(3): 193–211.

41 Hofstede G (1980) *Culture's Consequences*. SAGE Publications, London.

42 Trompenaars F and Hampden-Turner C (1997) *Riding the Waves of Culture: understanding cultural diversity in business*. Nicholas Brealey Publishing Ltd, London.

43 Buijs G (1996) *Migrant Women: crossing boundaries and changing identities.* Berg, Oxford.

44 Rogaly B (1999) Poverty and social exclusion in Britain: where finance fits. In: B Rogaly, T Fisher and E Mayo (1999) *Poverty, Social Exclusion and Microfinance in Britain.* Oxfam GB and the New Economics Foundation, Oxford.

45 De Foucauld JB and Piveteau D (1995) *La Société en quête de sens.* Odile Jacob, Paris. http://216.239.59.104/search?q-=cache:P1Omk-YdcxQJ:www.phac-aspc.gc.ca/ph-sp/phdd/news2001/pdf/social_exclusion_en.pdf+De+Foucauld.+J.+B.+and+Piveteau.+D.+(1995)+&hl=en&ie=UTF-8

46 Narayan D, Chambers R, Shah MK *et al.* (2000) *Voices of the Poor, Crying Out for Change.* Oxford University Press, Oxford.

47 Sen A (2000) *Social Exclusion: concept, application, and scrutiny.* Social Development Papers No 1. Office of Environment and Social Development, Asian Development Bank.

48 Lau DC and Murnighan JK (1998) Demographic diversity and faultlines: the compositional dynamics of organisational groups. *Academy of Management Review.* **23**(2): 325–40.

49 Harrison DA, Price KH and Bell MP (1998) Beyond relational demography: time and the effects of surface- and deep-level diversity on work group cohesion. *Academy of Management Journal.* **41**(1): 96–107.

50 Suter E (1997) *Employment Law Checklist.* Institute of Personnel and Development, London.

51 Lewis D (1998) *Essentials of Employment Law.* Institute of Personnel and Development, London.

52 DH (2000) *The Vital Connection: an equalities framework for the NHS.* Department of Health, London.

53 Phoenix A (2002) A monocultural nation in a multi-cultural society? British continuities and discontinuities in the racialised and gendered nation. In: I Lenz, H Lutz, M Morokvasic-Müller *et al.* (ed) *Crossing Borders and Shifting Boundaries. Vol. 2: Gender, Identities and Networks.* Leske and Budrich, Opladen, Germany.

54 Khan (1991) *Ethnicity in the 1991 Census. Annual Local Area Labour Force Survey Vol. 4. October 2001.* The Stationary Office, Office for National Statistics, London. www.statistics.gov.uk/STATBASE/ssdataset.asp?vlnk=6282.

55 Eversley J and Watts H (2001) *Refugee and Overseas Qualified Nurses Living in the UK.* Praxis and Queen Mary and Westfield, University of London, London.

56 McKay S and Winkelmann-Gleed A (2005) *Migrant Workers in the East of England, draft report.* WLRI, London Metropolitan University and EEDA, London.

57 CRE (2002) www.cre.gov.uk/duty/ethnicmonitoring.html.

58 Culley L and Dyson S (2001) *Ethnicity and Nursing Practice.* Palgrave, Basingstoke.

59 Davies C (1995) *Gender and the Professional Predicament in Nursing.* Open University Press, Buckingham.

60 Davies J (2002) Strong-arm tactics. *Health Service Journal.* **21 November:** 24–7.

61 Ekstrom DN (1999) Gender and perceived nurse caring in nurse-patient dyads. *Journal of Advanced Nursing.* **29**(6): 1393–401.

62 Evans JA (2002) Cautious caregivers: gender stereotypes and the sexualisation of men nurses' touch. *Journal of Advanced Nursing.* **40**(4): 441–8.

63 Fealy GM (2004) 'The good nurse': visions and values in images of the nurse. *Journal of Advanced Nursing.* **46**(6): 649–56.

64 Whittock M, Edwards C, McLaren S *et al.* (2002) 'The tender trap': gender, part-time nursing and the effects of 'family friendly' policies on career advancement. *Sociology of Health and Illness.* **24**(3): 305–26.

65 Muldoon O and Reilly J (2003) Career choice in nursing students: gendered constructs as psychological barriers. *Journal of Advanced Nursing.* **43**(1): 93–100.

66 de Lange T (2004) *Nurses are single, doctors have wives? Gender bias in Dutch regulation of labour migration, 1945–2005.* Paper presented at the Gendered Borders Conference, Vrije Universtiteit, Amsterdam, 30 September–2 October 2004. Available at www. rechten. vu.nl/dbfilestream.asp?id=1476 (accessed 16 October 2004).

67 Evans JA (2004) Men nurses: a historical and feminist perspective. *Journal of Advanced Nursing.* **47**(3): 321–8.

68 Öhlén J and Segesten K (1998) The Professional Identity of the Nurse: Concept Analysis and Development. *Journal of Advanced Nursing.* **28**(4): 720–7.

69 Leonard P (2003) 'Playing' doctors and nurses? Competing discourse of gender, power and identity in the British National Health Service. *The Sociological Review.* **51**(2): 219–37.

70 Williams CL (1995) Hidden advantages for men in nursing. *Nursing Administration Quarterly.* **19**(2): 63–70.

71 MacDougall G (1997) 'Caring a masculine perspective'. *Journal of Advanced Nursing.* **25**: 809–13.

72 Hearn J (1982) Notes on patriarchy, professionalization and semi-professions. *Sociology.* **16**: 184–202.

73 Charles N (2002) *Gender in Modern Britain.* Oxford University Press, Oxford.

74 Connell RW (1987) *Gender and Power.* Polity Press, Cambridge.

75 Mackintosh M (1981) Gender and economics, the sexual division of labour and the subordination of women. In: K Young, C Wolkowitz and R McCullagh (ed) *Of Marriage and the Market: women's subordination in international perspective.* CSE Books, London.

76 Moore HL (1994) *A Passion for Difference: essays in anthropology and gender.* Blackwell Publishers Ltd, Oxford.

77 McNay L (2000) *Gender and Agency: reconfiguring the subject in feminist and social theory.* Polity Press, Cambridge.

78 Mohanty CT (1991) Under western eyes, feminist scholarship and colonial discourses. In: CT Mohanty, A Russo and L Torres (ed) *Third World Women and the politics of feminism.* Indiana University Press, Bloomington.

79 Young K, Wolkowitz C and McCullagh R (1981) *Of Marriage and the Market: women's subordination in international perspective*. CSE Books, London.

80 The Nursing and Midwifery Council (2004) *Statistical Analysis of the Register 1 April 2002 to 31 March 2003*. www.nmc-uk.org/nmc/main/publications/annualstatistics 2002–2003.pdf (accessed 16 October 2004).

81 RCN (2004) *A Report from the RCN Refugee Nurses Database, September 2004*. Royal College of Nursing and Midwifery, London.

82 Anderson P (2005). Men in a women's world. www.justfornurses.co.uk/career/ careerpath/Meninawomen.htm (accessed 18. April 2005).

83 Porter S (1992) Women in a women's job: the gendered experience of nurses. *Sociology of Health & Illness*. **14**(4): 510–27.

84 Summerfield H (1996) Patterns of adaptation: Somali and Bangladeshi women in Britain. In: G Buijs (ed), *Migrant Women: crossing boundaries and changing identities*. Berg, Oxford.

85 Bhachu P (1993) Identities constructed and reconstructed: representations of Asian women in Britain. In G Buijs (ed) *Migrant Women: crossing boundaries and changing identities*. Berg, Oxford.

86 Labour Force Survey (2000) *Managerial Responsibility of Employees: by gender and ethnic group, Spring 2000*. Office of National Statistics, London. http:/www.statistics. gov.uk/STATBASE/Expodata/Spreadsheets/D3475.xls

87 Berkowitz N (2000) *Gender Guidelines for the UK: forced migration review*. Refugee Studies Centre, Oxford.

88 Harzig C (2003) Immigration policies: a gendered historical comparison. In: M Morokvasic-Müller, U Erel and K Shinozaki (ed) *Crossing Borders and Shifting Boundaries. Vol 1: Gender on the Move*. Leske and Budrich, Opladen, Germany.

89 Nkomo SM (1988) Race and Sex: the forgotten case of the Black female manager. In S Rose and L Larwood (ed) *Women's Careers: pathways and pitfalls*. Praeger, New York.

90 Ely RJ (1994) The effects of organizational demographics and social identity on relationships among professional women. *Administrative Science Quarterly*. **39**: 203–38.

91 Williams JA and Giles H (1978) The changing status of women in society: an intergroup perspective. In: H Tajfel (ed.) *Differentiation Between Social Groups*. Academic Press, London.

92 Parrenas RS (2001) *Servants of Globalisation: women, migration and domestic work*. Stanford University Press, Stanford.

93 Rogaly B (1998) Workers on the move, seasonal migration and changing social relations in rural India. *Gender and Development*. **6**(1): 21–9.

94 Bock G and James S (1992) *Beyond Equality and Difference: citizenship, feminist politics, female subjectivity*. Routledge, London.

CHAPTER 3

The case of migrant nurses

Labour deficits in healthcare capacity

With the persistent shortage of nursing staff in the NHS, healthcare employment is closely linked to migrant labourers[1] and it has to be noted that the literature on the employment of UK residents from Black and minority ethnic backgrounds does not distinguish between motives for immigration, thus working immigrants, migrants and refugees are all placed in the same category of Black and minority ethnic workers.[2-6] Nurses' recruitment from overseas declined in the 1970s as a result of changes in immigration law and by the mid-1980s it was negligible. Since then the United States and Canada have become major destinations for skilled migrants.[7] Over recent years, though, the British government is seeking to increase its healthcare capacity[8] through major international recruitment efforts[9-10] and many of these focus, as noted above, on recruiting nurses directly from countries such as the Philippines, South Africa and India.[11-13] Such labour migration has long-term repercussions for the countries of origin, the so-called 'brain drain'. For example, Jamaica has lost so many nurses that it had to resort to the recruitment of Cuban nurses. Clearly, international recruitment of foreign workers can hamper domestic supply.

Such attempts to address acute staffing problems have been much in the news in recent years. The BBC, for example, reported on 6 January 1999 that 'hospital managers have had to recruit nurses from South Africa in a bid to stave off a staffing crisis'[14] while Brindle, writing in the *Guardian* (17 May 2000) said that 'the NHS is turning to China in a desperate attempt to recruit nurses for Britain's short-staffed hospitals'.[15] This exodus of nursing staff in search of better paid opportunities in the UK has not gone without comment, not least because of the stress falling numbers of qualified staff puts on health services in the home country.[16] However, the quest for qualified nursing staff shows no sign of abating. Sawer[17] writing in the *Evening Standard* on 9 July suggested that 'Refugees and minorities can solve NHS staff crisis'. Indeed, skilled refugees in search of a better life would seem to offer a pool of potential NHS employees:

Africa sometimes appears a continent packed with people wanting to escape. The reasons are elementary: schools without chalk, hospitals without drugs, homes without food. And, in places such as Somalia, ravaged by war, countries without leaders. In comparison, the West holds at least the promise of a better life ... The ways out are official, unofficial and plain desperate.[18]

Thousands of nurses have been 'imported' from the Philippines, which has no historic links with Britain. Others have come from South Africa, India or Australia. An estimate from the Labour Force Survey (1988–90) concludes that in the late 1980s about 8% of all employed nurses were from minority ethnic backgrounds.[19] The best source is data collected by the Nursing and Midwifery Council on Non-EU and EU admissions to the register, which shows a dramatic increase since the late 1990s.[20] Currently there are around 30 000 non-British-trained nurses working in the NHS. Out of these only between 1200 and 1400 nurses per year have registered from other EU countries since 1998. Current figures from the Nursing and Midwifery Council showed that in 2001/2 nearly half of all new nurses on the register were from abroad (over 16 000 in total), originating mainly in the Philippines, Africa and Australia. This led the TUC to estimate that nearly half of all London-based nurses (47%) had come to Britain as migrants.[21]

Ball *et al.*[22] found that 3% of UK nurses are trained overseas, compared to 13% in London. In some London-based Trusts the overseas-trained workforce constitutes between 12–25% of the total qualified nursing workforce.

The Nursing and Midwifery Council's overseas registration statistics show a steady increase in the number of nurses and midwives being recruited from outside the UK and the European Community,[23–24] with the largest numbers in 2000/01, 2001/02 and 2002/03 coming from The Philippines, India and South Africa. It is often argued that some countries, like the Philippines, train a surplus of nurses in the assumption that many will work elsewhere and send remittances. Yet the number of nurses in the Philippines per 100 000 people is only half that of Britain.[25]

Recruitment from South Africa has led to an appeal by Nelson Mandela to stop Britain draining the country's medical staff.[26] Subsequently the Department of Health imposed a ban on recruitment from developing countries.[27] Nevertheless, due to independent migration and ongoing recruitment by private agencies, numbers of nurses from African countries working in Britain continue to rise. This trend highlights the complexity of regulating international recruitment and migration and the moral dilemma it involves.

This exodus of nursing staff from their home countries in search of better paid opportunities in the UK has not gone without comment, not least because of the stress falling numbers of qualified staff puts on health services in their home country. For example, Tobago and Trinidad lost one hundred of their psychiatric nurses to British hospitals, leaving them so drained of expertise that

Table 3.1   Initial Nursing and Midwifery Council (NMC) overseas admission to the register by country[23,24,39]

Country	1998/99	1999/00	2000/01	2001/02	2002/03	2003/04	2004/05
Philippines	52	1 052	3 396	7 235	5 594	4 338	2 521
India	30	96	289	994	1 833	3 073	3 690
South Africa	599	1 460	1 086	2 114	1 480	1 689	933
Australia	1 335	1 209	1 046	1 342	940	1 326	981
Nigeria	179	208	347	432	524	511	466
Zimbabwe	52	21	382	473	493	391	311
New Zealand	527	461	393	443	292	348	289
Ghana	40	74	140	195	255	354	272
Pakistan	3	13	44	207	172	140	205
Kenya	19	29	50	155	152	146	99
Zambia	15	40	88	183	135	169	162
USA	139	168	147	122	89	141	105
Mauritius	6	15	41	62	60	95	102
West Indies	221	425	261	248	57	397	352
Malawi	1	15	45	75	57	64	52
Canada	196	130	89	79	53	89	88
Botswana	4	–	87	100	42	90	91
Malaysia	6	52	34	33	27	24	
Singapore	13	47	48	43	25		
Jordan	3	3	33	49	18		
Others	128	427	357	478	649	737	697
Total	3 568	5 945	8403	15 062	12 947	14 122	11 416

units had to be closed. However, the quest for qualified nursing staff shows no sign of abating.

Table 3.1 shows seven years of overseas registration statistics for the leading countries from which nurses and midwives are being recruited. These do not include nurses and midwives trained within the European Union.

Most internationally qualified nurses are voluntary migrants who, unlike other groups of economic migrants, are welcomed due to the high number of nursing vacancies. Despite this seemingly warm reception, the integration of these nurses can be affected by the existing negative public attitude towards migrants and by the day-to-day employment conditions some of them meet.

Most migrant nurses from less developed countries start at the very bottom of the pay scale once they become registered nurses in Britain, regardless of their previous experience, length of service or speciality. Existing studies suggest that 'overseas' nurses are under-represented in senior grades, denied career progression and kept in auxiliary positions and less desirable clinical specialities. Moreover, there are reports of extensive discrimination on a personal and institutional level, leading to wide-ranging racial inequality.[28,29] With a shortage of suitably qualified nurses, migrant nurses have made a substantial professional contribution to the NHS, as described by Buchan[30] and Allan and Aggergaard Larsen.[31] Nevertheless, the examples of the lack of their integration into the workplace are symbolic of experiences of migrants in other professions.

The British healthcare system

The National Health Service was set up just over 50 years ago and is now, with one million employed staff, the largest employer in the UK. In England the NHS employs 782 100 staff members in total and out of these 338 600 are nurses, midwives and health visitors.[32] In London the NHS employs 55 000 nurses and midwives and requires an increase of 30% over the next five years to meet staffing requirements as a result of turnover and recruitment problems caused largely by the high costs of living in London.[33]

The figure below describes in very basic terms the NHS structure in England since April 2002. The Department of Health (DH), currently supported by eight regional offices, is responsible for health and personal social services in England, which includes oversight of the NHS. Currently 28 strategic health authorities provide strategic leadership of the NHS in their area. For example,

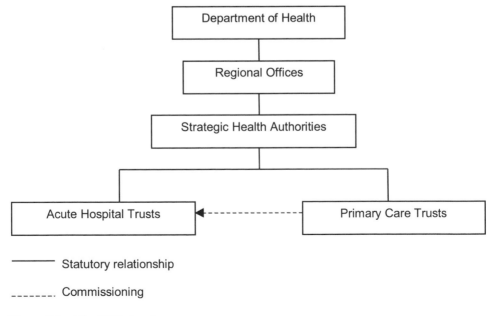

Figure 3.1   The NHS structure.

guidelines for the recruitment of internationally qualified nurses from certain countries or equal opportunities policies in line with legislation are published by the Department of Health and are binding for NHS Trusts.

NHS Trusts, established in 1991, are self-governing organisations with their own board of directors. Trusts are expected to make decisions about the strategic direction of the organisation, including staff recruitment and employment. primary care trusts were established in April 2000 and are responsible for the development of health services in the community, including general practitioners' services and the delivery of non-acute care services.

Hospital star ratings were introduced by the Department of Health in September 2001 to assess the performance of acute hospital trusts. Highest scoring hospitals are awarded three stars and lowest none. Even though highly controversial and currently under review, the system was extended to all NHS organisations in 2002–2003 and reported indicators are:

1 **clinical focus:** inpatient waiting, clinical negligence, outpatient waiting, emergency readmission, long inpatient waits, deaths in hospital, breast cancer waits, financial performance
2 **patient focus:** 12-hour trolley waits, inpatient waiting, cancelled operations, outpatient waiting, treatment of staff, 4-hour trolley waits, hospital cleanliness, complaints resolved
3 **staff focus:** sickness, absence, junior doctors hours, consultant vacancies, nurse vacancies, allied health professional vacancies.

On a national level the NHS faces recruitment and retention problems, and is under financial strain. The NHS Plan for England, published by the Department of Health in July 2000, sets out a 10-year action plan to improve the services. It consists of five key objectives:

- improving health outcomes for everyone
- improving patient and carer experience of the NHS and social services
- effective delivery of appropriate care
- fair access
- value for money.

Amongst other targets the plan promises 7500 more consultants, 2000 additional GPs, and 20 000 additional nurses by the year 2005. The plan goes on to state that these targets will be achieved through recruitment, provision of training places and attracting back nurses who have left the profession. There are other promises, such as the improvement of working lives, pay structures and management on hospital wards.

In a White Paper the British government outlines a 10-year plan to reform the NHS into a 'health service provider fit for the 21st century'.[34] There is an urgent need to increase staff capacity in the NHS, which currently has around 10 000 vacancies for nurses, midwives and health visitors, of which 2 750 are in London.[35,36]

As a result of international recruitment one in three registered nurses in London is from overseas compared with the national average of one in ten.[37] Yet a considerable number of trained and experienced healthcare workers have either found refuge in Britain or have migrated to Britain for non-work-related reasons and some are seeking employment as part of their integration into society. With the current recruitment and retention problems in Britain's healthcare sector, one would assume that particular efforts are being made to attract such nurses into the existing workforce.[38] However, only a few employers have taken the initiative in supporting refugee nurses, others who migrated independently of recruitment agencies and nurses who were recruited to work in Care Homes but hold extensive nursing skills. Thus these migrant nurses still present an underused resource for the NHS.

The process of nurses' registration in Britain

Nursing, midwifery and health visiting has its own statutory body in the UK, namely the Nursing and Midwifery Council (NMC). This council develops and monitors professional standards for nurses, midwives and health visitors and maintains a register of individuals trained in these professions. Thus all migrant nurses wanting to work in the NHS, as well as in the independent healthcare sector, need firstly to register with the NMC.

Table 3.2 Non-UK trained nurses: initial registration with the NMC[30,39]

Year	Trained in EU countries	Trained in other countries	Total non-UK trained
1994/95	798	1 654	2 452
1995/96	763	1 999	2 762
1996/97	1 141	2 633	3 774
1997/98	1 439	2 861	4 300
1998/99	1 412	3 568	4 980
1999/00	1 416	5 945	7 361
2000/01	1 291	8 403	9 694
2001/02 (estimated)	1 093	15 062	16 155
2002/03	836	12 947	13 783
2003/04	1 030	14 122	15 152
2004/05	1 193	11 416	12 609
	12 412	80 610	93 022

As Table 3.1 above has shown, there is a significant increase in the number of migrant nurses initially registering in the UK since the late 1990s and, as Table 3.2 shows, most of these are from non-EU countries.

These figures contain nurses directly recruited into UK employment as well as those who came to Britain for other reasons, such as refugees. This lack of distinction by the Nursing and Midwifery Council can cause confusion because it amalgamates 'ethically' and 'unethically' (according to or in breach of DH recruitment guidelines) recruited nurses, refugees and others trained outside the UK into the same category. This can lead to misleading conclusions in the analysis as to where nurses are coming from and why they are here in Britain.

Qualifications of fully trained nurses from EU countries are accepted as part of inter-government agreements among EU member states. However, migrants belonging to the latter group need to apply to the Nursing and Midwifery Council to have their training and professional experience verified. Therefore all non-EU nurses need to pass an International English Language Testing System (IELTS), need to provide written evidence of their qualifications and need to provide written references. International English Language Testing System is not a requirement for nurses from EU countries, even though they may have limited English language comprehension and communication skills too. The Nursing and Midwifery Council then considers this evidence provided by migrant nurses and either advises the nurse to apply for a supervised practice placement for a period generally between 3–12 months, or refuses their application. If accepted, the nurse then has to find a hospital that provides a placement relevant to the experience required by the Nursing and Midwifery Council.

The process in itself provides a number of hurdles for non-EU trained nurses, including those who came as refugees. First, getting information about the procedure itself may be difficult; second, passing a language test poses a challenge for non-English speakers and there are concerns that the IELTS test is not the best method of assessing migrant nurses' communication skills. In addition, a fee of £117 needs to be paid by the individual in order to have their application processed and a further fee of £93 is due once the application for registration has been accepted. The registration is reviewed every three years and in order to keep it alive, the fee of £93 has to be paid every three years. Only for those internationally qualified nurses who can provide evidence of their refugee status may the first payment be waived. To some this might be seen as giving refugees preferential treatment compared to other migrant nurses, but the process is so arduous that some refugee nurses have found it easier to pay. Third, original identity and qualification documents have to be presented to the Nursing and Midwifery Council[40–42] and past professional experience has to be supported by references from previous employers. This disadvantages refugees and asylum seekers who often fled without documents and may find it hard to obtain previous employment references if they left for political reasons or come from war-torn countries. Fourth, internationally qualified nurses have to provide evidence of their immigration status and right to work in Britain. For the sub-group of refugees, a key axis for comparison in the research, this means providing a copy of the Home Office decision and a social security support letter.

In comparison, for internationally qualified nurses who are directly recruited by NHS Trusts much of this registration process is done by a recruitment agency. Migrant nurses are also recruited by the independent healthcare sector in Britain, which has similar written guidelines to those issued by the Department of Health for the NHS in order to prevent unfair treatment of nurses. However, these principles are not compulsory and there are many examples of private hospitals and care homes not complying with best practice and continuing to recruit internationally qualified nurses from developing countries facing an acute shortage in their medical workforce.[43]

The nurses who are directly recruited receive their work permit through the hospital, and the decision by the Nursing and Midwifery Council and their placement are sorted out before they arrive in the UK.[44,45] In contrast, migrant nurses who came to Britain independently must take individual initiative through this multi-staged procedure in order to progress into healthcare employment. This is an important distinction between independent migrants/ refugees and directly internationally recruited nurses. The Nursing and Midwifery Council then compares professional nursing qualifications from different countries with the standards required in Britain.

Organisational changes, including changes to the information technology (IT) system and a name change from the United Kingdom Council for Nurses and Midwives (UKCC) to the current name, Nursing and Midwifery Council (NMC), in April 2002, led to delays in processing applications to the register. However, an internal review of the application process by the Council has now achieved a more efficient and speedy procedure.

Once a positive reply has been received from the Nursing and Midwifery Council, finding a supervision placement takes yet more time, as they are in short supply, partially due to a shortage of suitable mentors. Consequently the process of having their skills recognised in Britain is a long-winded procedure which can potentially lead to frustration and despair.

Regardless of their reasons for migration (fleeing persecution or political unrest, wanting to gain work experience or English language skills, marriage or other personal relationships or economic reasons), similar issues are faced by all migrant nurses regarding their professional integration. These include having to comply with regulatory bodies, having to get used to a new organisational structure, and sorting out finances and commitments to family members. For refugees this process further adds to their uncertainties: there may be insecurity about the well-being of family members who were left behind, certificates and employment references may be missing or be unobtainable, and the immigration status may still be temporary. Examples of personal experiences are synthesised in subsequent sections of this and following chapters.

Of relevance to migrants' integration and their contribution to organisational capacity are the following important distinctions between the different sub-groups of non-UK trained nurses:

1 internationally trained in the EU
2 internationally trained outside EU and directly recruited from abroad
3 internationally trained outside EU and independent migrant
4 internationally trained outside EU and asylum seeker/refugee.

These distinctions have direct relevance for the individual nurse's pathway through the registration procedures with its impact on:

- motivation, frustration and perceptions of fairness
- job satisfaction
- work-related identities
- ability to commit to an organisation and identify with what it stands for.

Current studies on nurses who migrated independently of recruitment agencies to Britain are mainly limited to papers on the barriers met by this group of nurses when trying to gain access to employment.[46-50] Refugee-specific barriers consist of lack of ability to speak and comprehend English, access to professional documents to prove past qualifications and work experience and access to work references. A lack of guidance and encouragement from employers and regulatory bodies as to how past qualifications can be recognised in Britain has also been reported.[51,52] Employment is strongly viewed as a stepping-stone in the integration process and this book examines the process of integration through the individual nurses' perceptions of their organisation, colleagues and supervisors and their reported work-related feelings.

An empirical study

Methodologically sections of this book are based on empirical research carried out in 2002/03, combining a self-reported survey, measuring organisational attitudes and employee well-being, and in-depth interviews, drawing on individual experiences of workplace integration. This combination of personal testimony and quantitative data analysis, explained further below, merges the strengths of both methods.

Semi-structured in-depth interviews

The focus of the empirical analysis was on migrant nurses who came to Britain independently of recruitment agencies, including asylum seekers and refugees.

Their integration into British health sector employment was researched by looking at individuals' workplace experiences through their own eyes. This was done by interviewing a sample of 22 migrant nurses, including refugees. Some of them were re-interviewed two or three times, in order to gain a longitudinal picture of their integration and how they progressed as nurses into employment. The sample was generated through access to a database owned by Praxis Community Projects Ltd. Praxis offers individual support, lobbys with regulatory bodies, key managers in the NHS and other stakeholders; and provides 'pre-adaptation courses', which offer an introduction to the British healthcare system and prepare internationally qualified nurses for their supervised practice placements. At the time of the research the participants fulfilled the following criteria:

- they had completed the necessary language and other requirements set by the Nursing and Midwifery Council and
- they were either undertaking their supervision placement or
- they were fully employed in the British healthcare sector.

Self-administered survey

A self-administered survey (n = 358) was introduced at five London-based hospitals with between 6% and 53.5% of their nursing workforce being internationally qualified. This represented 4.02% of internationally qualified nurses in London.

The same key objectives informed the design of the survey, which was distributed to a wider group of migrant nurses, including internationally recruited nurses employed by the participating hospitals. The hospitals were selected partly through self-selection and partly through personal contacts or because of the hospital's initiatives in recruiting internationally qualified and refugee nurses. The hospitals include four NHS Trusts and a small private hospital.

The quantitative and qualitative data cover the same themes. The semi-structured interviews also informed the open-ended questions in the survey, which were used in addition to the quantitative Likert scales to offer scope for the expression of explanations and examples. The application of validated measures in the survey means that the results were not dependent on the researcher and if the survey were to be conducted by someone else the outcomes should be unchanged.

The survey consisted of:

1   a number of previously tested measures[53] using a seven-point Likert scale and
2   related open-ended questions, which gave respondents the opportunity to elaborate on issues such as 'welcome by the hospital', 'job satisfaction',

'feelings about career development at the hospital', 'support received by the mentor', 'overall perception of treatment', 'personal contribution' and space for further comments. Thus respondents could expand on reasons, give examples and verbalise opinion. A further open-ended question was included in the section on 'ethnicity'. Here the 2001 census categories were used and in addition the respondent was offered the opportunity to self-define their ethnicity if they could not identify with any of the given categories.

The survey comprised three main sections, A, B and C.

- Section A covered background information, such as job title, current and previous speciality, employment tenure, working hours and shift patterns.
- Section B covered first, work-related factors (organisational effectiveness, involvement, promotion opportunity, supervisory and peer support, fairness at work, innovation and equal opportunities) and second, work attitudes (job satisfaction, intention to stay with the organisation, different types of commitment emotions).
- Section C asked questions about more personal information, such as age, gender, reason for coming to Britain, ethnicity, marital status, number of dependents and financial support sent outside UK.

A response rate of 38% was achieved and thus the total sample of completed and useable returned surveys was (n = 140).

Table 3.3 provides an overview of the demographic characteristics of the survey sample, referred to in subsequent chapters.

With the mean *age* of the sample being 34 years, the youngest respondent was 22 and the oldest was 59. The median age was 32 years, and more than half of the sample (51%) was under the age of 32. This is significant, as the average age of the nursing population is rising and nearly half of NHS nurses and midwives are over 40, with the number of retirements rising.[54] Most survey respondents had worked in their current post and for their current employer for less than 2 years, even though the average internationally trained nurse had 10 years' nursing experience. This potentially raises concerns about turnover rates.

Looking at the survey data on 'ethnicity' confirms that a large number of Filipino nurses were employed by the participating trusts, most of whom had been directly recruited from the Philippines. Currently, nearly half of all new nurses on the national register are from abroad, again confirming concerns about turnover, particularly in London, where the cost of living is higher than in the rest of Britain. Only 12% of survey respondents reported that they migrated to Britain for economic reasons, although two-thirds were sending money to support family members outside Britain. Thus while salary levels may not have been the primary reported reason for migration, it certainly presented a strong motivation to work in Britain. The sample included 12 refugees or asylum seekers and this sub-group has been used in subsequent comparisons.

Table 3.3 Demographic description of the survey sample

Measure		Total percentages (rounded up or down)
Number of respondents		n = 140
Demographic means	Age in years	34.19
Gender	Male	17.9%
	Female	82.1%
Ethnicity	White	2.9%
	Mixed	62.1%
	Asian, including Filipino	20.7%
	Black	1.4%
	Chinese	12.9%
Marital status	Single	40%
	Living together	1.4%
	Married	46.4%
	Widowed	4.3%
	Separated/divorced	7.9%
Dependants in UK	Yes (not reported 18.6%)	35%
	No	46.4%
Hours worked	Full-time	97.9%
	Part-time	2.1%
Financial support to relatives outside UK	Yes	75.7%
	No	24.3%

Key informants

Key informant interviews with NHS Hospital Trust managers and individuals involved in the recruitment and integration of migrant nurses were undertaken. This allows for comparison between their perception of workplace integration and contributions made by migrant nurses to the organisation with those shared by the individual nurses.

Migrant nurses in London

The primary criteria for the selection of London as a research site was:

1   the accessibility to migrants and more specifically to refugee nurses already in employment or on a supervision programme in the NHS and

2   the high vacancy rate for all NHS posts, which remains far higher in London than elsewhere in Britain.[55]

As a result of contacting stakeholders working with migrant nurses who migrated independently of recruitment agencies, it quickly became clear that in the year 2000 London was the only UK location with advanced programmes assisting such nurses to gain access to NHS employment. The main reasons given for other locations not running programmes for independent migrant nurses, including refugees, were lack of funding, lack of placements for supervision, institutional racism by hospitals towards this sub-group of migrants and difficulty in securing co-operation from the regulatory bodies.

There is no reliable information on the number of migrants or migrant nurses who came independently of recruitment agencies, but evidence shows that there are more in London than elsewhere in Britain.[56,57] This is mainly due to the high percentage of migrants concentrated in Greater London. A full 60% of all migrants live in South East England, with 42% living in London, compared to only 10% of the UK-born population living in London.[58] The total number of refugees and asylum seekers entering London over the past 15 years has been estimated to be between 240 000 and 280 000, with some boroughs having significantly higher numbers than others. Some of the boroughs with the highest percentage of residents born outside the EU are Newham (35.6%), Tower Hamlets (30.5%) and Hackney (29.5%).[59] In these boroughs some hospitals have been actively engaged in particularly giving refugee nurses access to employment.

References

1   Culley L and Dyson S (2001) *Ethnicity and Nursing Practice*. Palgrave, Basingstoke.

2   Modood T, Berthoud R, Lakey J *et al.* (1997) *Ethnic Minorities in Britain, Diversity and Disadvantage*. Policy Studies Institute, London.

3   Panayi P (1999) *The Impact of Immigration: a documentary history of the effects and experiences of immigrants in Britain since 1945*. Manchester University Press, Manchester.

4   Parekh B (2000) *The Future of Multi-ethnic Britain: the Parekh report*. The Runnymede Trust, London.

5   Parekh B (2000) *Rethinking Multiculturalism: cultural diversity and political theory*. Macmillan Press, London.

6   Ramdin R (1999) *Reimaging Britain: 500 Years of Black and Asian history*. Pluto Press, London.

7   ILO (2003) Skilled labour mobility: review of issues and evidence. In: Japan Institute of Labour (ed) *Migration and the Labour Market in Asia: recent trends and policies*. OECD, Paris.

8 NHS (2001) *Guidance for the Provision of Supervised Practice for Nurses and Adaptation for Midwives in London.* NHS London Regional Office, London.

9 DH (2001) *Code of Practice for NHS Employers.* Department of Health, London.

10 DH (2001) *Review Body for Nursing Staff, Midwives, Health Visitors and Professions Allied to Medicine, Review for 2002.* Department of Health with written evidence from the health departments for Great Britain, London.

11 Carr-Brown J (2002) Quarter of nurses come from abroad. *Sunday Times.* **9 June**: 2.

12 Buchan J (2000) *Abroad Minded.* Queen Margaret University College, Edinburgh.

13 Laurance J (2003) Nurses from abroad still lured to UK despite ban. *The Independent.* **12 May**: 5.

14 BBC News (1999) Health Hospital recruits South African nurses. http://news.bbc. co.uk/l/hi/health/249619.stm (accessed May 2004).

15 Brindle D (2000) Hospitals look to China to ease nurses crisis: the future of the NHS: special report. *The Guardian.* **17 May**: 7.

16 Ray M (2001) Brain drain to hit SA growth. *The Cape Times.* **6 June**: 1. www.iol.co.za/ general/news/newsprint.php?art_id=ct20010606212513149S420318&sf=

17 Sawer P (2003) Refugees and minorities 'can solve NHS staff crisis'. *Evening Standard.* **9 July**: 15.

18 Walsh D (2003) Desperate journeys to escape homelands without hope. *The Independent.* **19 June**: 4.

19 Beishon S, Virdee S and Hagell A (1995) *Nursing in a Multi-ethnic NHS.* Policy Studies Institute, London.

20 Buchan J (2002) *The International Recruitment of Nurses: United Kingdom Case Study: 28.* Royal College of Nursing, Queen Margaret University College, Edinburgh.

21 TUC (2002) *Migrant Workers: a TUC guide.* TUC and JCWI, London.

22 Ball J and Pike G (2004) *Stepping Stones: results from the RCN membership survey 2003.* Royal College of Nursing, London. Available at www.rcn.org/publications/pdf/ membershipsurvey2003.pdf.

23 NMC (2004) *Recent overseas trained nurses and midwives registering with the NMC 'Top twenty'.* www.nmc-uk.org/nmc/main/pressStatements/recordNumberOfNurses FromIndiaToWorkInUk.html (accessed 2005).

24 NMC (2004) www.nmc-uk.org/nmc/main/advice/enrolledNursing.html (accessed 2005).

25 Aiken LH, Buchan J, Sochalski J *et al.* (2004) Trends in international nurse migration. *Health Affairs.* **23**(3): 69–77.

26 Carvel J, Butler P and Batty D (2003) NHS imports staff from South Africa to cut waiting lists. *The Guardian.* **12 February**: 13.

27 DH (1999) *Guidance on International Nursing Recruitment.* Department of Health, London.

28 Baxter C (1988) *The Black Nurse: an endangered species*. National Extension College, Cambridge.

29 Ellis B (1990) Racial equality: the nursing profession. The King's Fund, London.

30 Buchan J (2002) *The International Recruitment of Nurses: United Kingdom Case Study: 28*. Royal College of Nursing, Queen Margaret University College, Edinburgh.

31 Allan H and Aggergaard Larson J (2003) *We Need Respect: experiences of internationally recruited nurses in the UK*. Royal College of Nursing, London.

32 The NHS Confederation (2002) *The Pocket Guide to the NHS in England 2002*. The NHS Confederation, London.

33 Easmon C (2003) *Making it Happen in the NHS*. Paper presented at the Refugee Nurses into Employment Conference, London.

34 Foster A (2002) *The NHS Plan*. March 2003. Director of Human Resources for the NHS, London. Department of Health, London. www.dh.gov.uk/assetRoot/04/05/58/66/04055866.pdf

35 Laurance J (2002) Overseas NHS staff are delayed by red tape. *The Independent*. **11 March**: 6.

36 Laurance J (2003) Nurses from abroad still lured to UK despite ban, *The Independent*. **12 May**: 5.

37 Buchan J (2000) Abroad Minded. Queen Margaret University College, Edinburgh.

38 The Nursing Times (2002) Filipino nurses 'lack personal care skills'. *Nursing Times*. **98**(7): 5.

39 NMC (2005) New 2004/2005 statistics for nurses and midwives. **21 September**. http://www.nmc-uk.org/(qb0ivrr31jdhfu45p2zw1145)/aArticle.aspx?ArticleID=1792

40 NMC (2002) *Registering as a Nurse or Midwife in the United Kingdom*. Nursing and Midwifery Council, London.

41 NMC (2002) *Requirements for Pre-registration Nursing Programmes*. Nursing and Midwifery Council, London.

42 NMC (2002) *Fitness for Practice and Purpose*. Nursing and Midwifery Council, London.

43 UNISON (2001) *A UNISON Guide for Nurses from Overseas Working in the UK*. UNISON, London.

44 NHS (2001) *Guidance for the Provision of Supervised Practice for Nurses and Adaptation for Midwives in London*. NHS London Regional Office, London.

45 NHS (2002) *Employment Improves Your Health: regeneration and employment in health and social care*. NHS London Regional Office, Workforce and Development, London.

46 Coker N (2001) *Racism in Medicine: an agenda for change*. King's Fund Publishing, London.

47 Refugee Council (1999) *Creating the Conditions for Refugees to Find Work. A Report for the Refugee Council*. The British Refugee Council, London.

48 RCN (2001) *Welcome to the UK, Welcome to the RCN*. Royal College of Nursing, London.

49 Hardill I and MacDonald S (2000) Skilled international migration: the experience of nurses in the UK. *Regional Studies.* **34**(7): 681–92.

50 Harrison S (2003) White nurses dominate shortlists for senior ranks. *Nursing Standard.* **23**: 6.

51 Eversley J (1999) *The Reality is Different: interviews with the target group and beneficiaries of Pathways to Access Project.* Queen Mary and Westfield, University of London, PPRU, London.

52 Eversley J and Watts H (2001) *Refugee and Overseas Qualified Nurses Living in the UK.* Praxis and Queen Mary and Westfield, University of London, London.

53 Price JL (1997) Handbook of organizational measurement. *International Journal of Manpower, International Manpower Forecasting, Planning and Labour Economics.* **18**(4, 5, 6): 1–560.

54 Finlayson B, Dixon J, Meadows S *et al.* (2002) Mind the gap: the extent of the NHS nursing shortage. *BMJ.* **325**: 538–41.

55 Hutt R and Buchan J (2005) *Trends in London's NHS Workforce: an updated analysis of key data.* King's Fund, London.

56 Buchan JFB and Gouch P (2002) *In Capital Health? Meeting the challenges of London's health care workforce.* The King's Fund, London.

57 Bardsley M and Storkey M (2000) Estimating the number of refuges in London. *Journal of Public Health Medicine.* **22**(3): 406–12.

58 Haque R (2002) *Migrants in the UK: a descriptive analysis of their characteristics and labour market performance, based on the Labour Force Survey.* Department of Works and Pensions, Leeds.

59 Census data. www.statistics.gov.uk/census2001/default.asp.

Motivation to migrate and work

This book suggests that the success of migrants integrating into their workplace depends on aspects of personal and work-related *identities*, some of which become apparent through the individuals' relationships at work. These have to take the *motivation* to work, *commitment to the organisation* and the *management of diversity* into account. This is reflected in this and the following chapters. First, they highlight facets of the motivating factors linked to migration and work in Chapter 4. Second, explore the experiences of migrant workers' integration through their encounters with colleagues, mentors and supervisors at work (*see* Chapter 5) and then go on to look at further aspects about meeting 'others' (*see* Chapters 6 and 7) before considering the migrant worker within the organisational context (*see* Chapter 8). Third, drawn from this analysis the linkage between well-being at work and migrant nurses making a positive contribution to the organisation is considered, leading to recommendations for management approaches that allow individuals from a minority background to become part of the existing team (*see* Chapter 9). This challenges perceptions of migrants based on prejudice and discrimination and the outline contributes to a framework for cross-cultural work teams, including indicators for a successful integration process based on inclusion and equality. A summary section and recommendations for policy and practice are outlined in the final chapter, Chapter 10.

Motivation in context

Motivation is a state of mind, a preparedness to do something and *intrinsic motivation* stems from the expected pleasure of the activity itself rather than from its results and is based on self-administered rewards, such as feelings of satisfaction, competence, self-esteem and accomplishment, rather than on rewards distributed by an external agent.[1] The individuals' perception of the reward motivates them. In contrast *extrinsic motivation* derives from rewards distributed by others, outside the task itself and stresses tangible benefits provided by organisational managers such as promotion, praise, pay increases or fringe benefits.

Concepts and theories relevant to motivation have been developed over the last century, to name just a few, 'Equity Theory',[2] Maslow's 'Hierarchy of Needs'[3] and 'Expectancy Theory',[4] which led to Porter and Lawler's 'Motivation Model'.[5] These concepts help us to understand the motivational and managerial processes talked about in this book and are mainly concerned with the intrinsic aspects of the motivation process; the benefits that are perceived to be valuable by the individual employees, such as self-esteem, perception of equality, success or accomplishment. Thus they are not measurable in monetary terms and rely on individual values.[6,7]

Equity Theory helps to explain why individuals perceive some situations as unfair. It relates to a process and argues that the perception of unfairness in an organisational setting leads to tension and motivates the individual to act in order to resolve unfairness. A status of inequity exists when the ratio between rewards (pay, recognition) and effort (time, ideas and input) is unequal. Action to resolve this can include putting in less effort, parting from the organisation or even profession or leaving hard tasks for others to do. Thus employees, such as nurses who are not paid based on their performance but by grades, may not put in as much effort as they could, unless they are intrinsically motivated to do so.

Maslow distinguishes in his *'Hierarchy of Needs' theory* between drives, which are biological determinants of behaviour, and other motives, which are socially constructed and acquired needs. Aspects of this hierarchy of needs from the most basic ones to the emotional ones can relate to the journey that refugees might go through as they flee and then integrate into British employment and society. Therefore past experiences and needs of migrant nurses and British-qualified nurses may vary significantly. For example, most British-trained nurses have probably never had to worry about access to clean water, food and shelter. Yet within the employment context human needs form part of individual identity and affect the associated value of perceived rewards. Nussbaum[8] draws a similar distinction between 'basic' capabilities, with which one is born, and 'internal' capabilities, acquired throughout life. In her approach Nussbaum then goes on to point out external constraints or facilitators, which can encourage or hamper individuals' capability to work. Such effect of external constraints on motivational processes is referred to in the employment conditions and policies.

Vroom developed *Expectancy Theory*, which describes the process by which motives become desirable outcomes. Expectancy is the perceived probability that effort will lead to good performance, which in turn leads to valued outcomes such as praise from a supervisor, higher wages, promotion or friendship with co-workers. Thus an individual, by doing a good job, expects some form of second-level outcome, related to valued intrinsic and extrinsic rewards. This theory was further developed by Porter and Lawler, leading to the *Motivation Model*. This model goes beyond motivational forces, and considers performance as a precursor to job satisfaction. Effort is mediated by individual abilities and traits, and by the person's perception of their job role. Porter and Lawler view motivation, satisfaction and performance as separate variables and attempt to explain the complex relationship among them.

The different motivations that cause individuals to cross international borders to migrate indicate that there is also a wide spectrum of motivations, some of which are related to work. Migrants themselves are seldom given a voice to share their perspectives relating to aspects of migration and employment. Therefore this and the following chapters illustrate steps along the journey of migrants' integration into British employment from the migrants' own perspective, based on their stories.

Motivations to migrate

The attitudes of some White British-born citizens towards migrant nurses do not always reflect a balanced, informed view. For example, on a recent visit to a care home for the elderly, the author shared with some of the residents that she had been to a wedding party hosted by refugees from Africa. The response from an otherwise confused, frail and quiet little lady was sharp and clear: 'Send them home!' Yet most of the nurses caring for her at the home were not born in Britain and it is possible that there may also have been asylum seekers among them.

The previous sections have shown that migrants are originating from diverse backgrounds, with their countries of origin affecting their migration patterns as well as their reception and integration into life in another country. Likewise there is a range of different reasons for individuals to migrate and some of these are:

- historic links – migrants whose countries of origin have historic links with the UK
- family-related – partners, family members or friends working in Britain
- economic reasons linked to high unemployment in the country of origin – to earn more money than they could in their country of origin
- international recruitment – being directly recruited from another country to fill vacancies
- adventure – a desire for new experiences
- language – a desire to improve their knowledge of English
- work experience – a desire to improve career options by working in another country
- threats and persecution – experience of threats or persecution in their country of origin leading individuals to flee and seek asylum.

Table 4.1 shows some examples of reported reasons for coming to the UK based on the empirical study. This is by no means an exhaustive list and as it is

Table 4.1 Self-reported reason among migrant nurses for coming to Britain

	Examples of reasons for coming to Britain	Percentages
1	Refugee/asylum seeker	8.57%
2	International recruitment	41.43%
3	Family-related and marriage	2.14%
4	Economic reasons	12.14%
5	Improve English	3.57%
6	Work experience	22.86%
7	Other	2.86%
	Not reported	6.43%

based on one empirical study it is not representative of migrants in general. There can also be a discrepancy between 'official reasons for coming' and actual personal reasons. For example, someone may have been directly recruited to work in the UK, but their own primary reason for coming was economic, to gain work experience or improve their English. Only 12% of survey respondents directly reported that they came to Britain for economic reasons. However, two-thirds were later saying that they were sending money to support family members outside Britain and it can be concluded that the majority of directly recruited nurses, over 40% of the sample, had an economic motive. A total of 12 respondents said that they had come to Britain as refugees or asylum seekers.

There are also other reasons for migrants to come to live and work in a Western country either temporarily or permanently and some of these are explored further.

Historic links

Many of the migrant nurses coming to Britain are originating from countries that have historical, colonial links to the UK, such as the West Indies, India, Pakistan and Ghana (*see* Table 3.1). While they still had UK passports, migration to the UK was a common occurrence and there were established communities they could join up with. Therefore for many years there have been a substantial number of Nigerian, Caribbean and Ghanaian nurses working in Britain.

Even though they had freedom of movement, personal circumstances could overrule a technical freedom to travel and the following nurse from Ghana was prohibited from leaving her country and only felt free to travel after the death of her father. She then travelled to work in Nigeria, Saudi Arabia and finally the UK while her husband remained behind in Ghana. She was in her fifties and mentioned that her friends and relatives had also come to work in the UK some time ago:

I have a lot of friends here, a lot of nieces. Most of them came down when the UKCC regarded you as a fully qualified nurse. I didn't come down because my father didn't allow me to travel. I was the only girl and he didn't want me to go. It was not until he died that I started travelling.

Despite such personal obstacles related to family values and gender norms, Commonwealth citizens have enjoyed more freedom to travel to Britain and indeed many of them came to work in the NHS. When the Nursing and Midwifery Council introduced changes to the nursing training and abolished the 'enrolled nurse' 2-year-training course in 2000, many nurses who had not upgraded their qualifications in time found themselves stuck working as Health Care Assistants rather than as fully qualified nurses. While there were good reasons to abolish a two-tier nursing system as enrolled nurses felt abused and patronised within the profession, some migrant nurses are now stuck with a dilemma.[9] A 45-year-old female nurse from Ghana made this explicit, saying:

All I wanted to do is get a PIN number or get someone who helps me to get more qualified. It is sometimes frustrating because you know that you can do this. I have been qualified since 1981, so I have done so many things: doing transfusion, doing dressings, theatre care. So, now I am working as an auxiliary and cannot do these things. That is very frustrating. When I came to England I went straight to UKCC and I was told that the enrolled nurses register is closed. So, what I have to do is to get a job in the NHS to convert my qualification or to do a full 3-year-training to get more qualified.

Following the interview the above nurse produced a stack of photos from her time in Ghana where trained nurses wore their uniforms to weddings as a sign of occupational status and pride. In contrast to some Western countries, nursing is seen in Ghana as a prestigious profession and wearing their uniforms in public is a sign of the nurses' confidence and high level of self-esteem. Few British-trained nurses would display their professional pride in quite the same way and it must seem unfamiliar for some migrant nurses to realise that nursing is not viewed as a desirable career choice among many young people in Britain, a country whose healthcare system they were looking up to for many years.

In 1998 the BBC estimated that 24 000 enrolled nurses had left the profession.[10] Seccombe *et al.*[11] conducted a study about enrolled nurses and their perception of their future in nursing in the UK. While many enrolled nurses, British-trained and non-British-trained, wanted to convert their qualification in the 1990s, a shortage of placements or individuals' contentment with being 'just' enrolled nurses meant that an equal number did not convert their qualification. While it seems impossible to obtain an accurate number of enrolled nurses currently in Britain, a number of Schools for Health and Nursing studies are offering conversion courses for British qualified enrolled nurses, yet there only seems to be one course directed at internationally qualified enrolled nurses who have recently arrived as migrants.

Historical links also account for large-scale recruitment of nurses and doctors from the Indian subcontinent, the Caribbean and other African countries. While there is a growing recognition that this depletes some developing countries of their healthcare workforce, nurses from such places are still migrating to Britain and are still actively recruited by the NHS or independent sector. This becomes apparent when looking at the long list of recruitment agencies aiming to fill UK-based vacancies without much concern of those left behind.

Family-related and demographical reasons

Closely linked to historic reasons to migrate to Britain are family-related ones and for some migrants it is not uncommon to relocate the whole family to the UK from Ghana, Nigeria, the Indian subcontinent, the Caribbean or more recently from Portugal and Eastern Europe. Due to nursing being such a female-orientated profession, in the past it was common for 'female' nurses to follow their 'male' partners as dependants when they changed their career paths. The following 46-year-old nurse from Ghana did just that:

> I was working in Ghana before. My husband came here to work as Presbyterian minister, so my husband brought me here. I had to take a job and support the family back home.

With four out of five survey respondents being female it was confirmed that even on an international scale, nursing remains a 'female-orientated career' (*see* Table 3.3).

Nearly 50% of the survey respondents were married and 40% were single (*see* Table 3.3). Very few were living together. There is also a possibility that some nurses who were separated or divorced reported that they were 'single'. These findings confirm the diversity of the migrant labour force and migration is by no means confined to people who are not in a committed relationship.

Even though nowadays many female nurses migrate alone, relationships still form a strong motivator for people to cross international boundaries and they comprise relationships with friends, partners or wider family relationships. Others come to Britain in order to marry or have met a partner who either is UK-based or wants to live in the UK for a while. The following midwife in her 20s had come to Britain to get married, but things did not work out and she found herself struggling alone to establish herself in exile personally as well as professionally about a year later:

> I come here first to get married and my husband was here in Britain but I had some problems and got divorced and then I decided to be independent.

Age is probably another factor affecting migration, with the mean age of the survey sample being 34.19 years, the youngest respondent being 22 years and the oldest 59 years. The median age was 32 years and more than half of the sample (51%) was relatively young, under 32 years of age. While many of the directly recruited nurses were relatively young, those who came as asylum seekers or independent of recruitment agencies reflected a wider age range, with some of the refugee nurses in their 40s.

Similar findings were made in a study of migrant workers in the East of England,[12] which showed that many younger migrant workers came as singles and were more prepared to accept seasonal work in less well regulated sectors, while some older workers came with family members. This study also showed that some older workers originating from countries with high unemployment rates such as Portugal, Brazil and Eastern Europe had found it difficult to secure work once they had reached their mid-forties. Although in danger of it being an over-generalisation, younger migrant workers seem more likely to identify their decision to move to the UK for work as an 'adventure', whereas older migrant workers are more likely to see it as the only route to employment, as this 50-year-old Brazilian woman noted:

> I retired in Brazil at the age of 45 years old. I used to be a secretary, working in a steel industry. I worked for 27 years in the same company. In Brazil at 45 years of age we have no further chance of getting a job. I had knowledge and experience but no chance to get a job.

Economic reasons

By far the highest number of migrant nurses would state economic reasons for them coming to the UK and most internationally recruited nurses are economically motivated. In addition they may also view working in Britain as a positive move in developing their career as well as improving their English, sometimes with the view of going on to work in other English-speaking countries, such as the US.

The findings from the empirical study were interesting because when asked for their motive to come to Britain, only 12% of respondents reported that they came for economic reasons, yet as many as two-thirds of the same sample reported that they were sending money to support family members outside Britain (*see* Table 3.3).

While the economic contributions that migrants are making to the British economy are being measured at about £2.4 billion,[13] economic reasons for migrations indicate a two-way-exchange. In addition to gaining financially, receiving organisations are benefiting from the skills and professional expertise migrants are contributing, and at the same time earning a salary enables them to provide financially for their families, who are often left behind.

Work experience and adventure

Young migrants often follow in the footsteps of their friends and may decide to work in another country for a while out of curiosity, adventurism or to develop their English language skills or career plans. For example, some agencies operating within agriculture or horticulture offer schemes for students from Eastern Europe to work in another country for just a season while continuing their studies. For nurses, however, such very short-term migration is rarely feasible due to the process for having their qualifications recognised in the UK. Yet nurses from EU member states or from Australia and New Zealand who do not need to go through a re-registration process tend to come to work in Britain for just a few months or years.

That is why international recruitment from other European countries, such as Scandinavia or Spain, is viewed as just a 'quick-fix' solution to the staffing needs of the British healthcare system. Very few of these nurses actually settle in the UK and NHS managers who tried recruiting from Western European countries confirmed that most nurses returned home within just a few years. Moreover, as they are not required to pass an English language test, but do not necessarily have a full grasp of the language, there are added communication barriers which are hard to address.

Thus for nurses from Canada, the US or Australia, working in Britain is viewed more as a 'gap-year' idea in the same way in which British citizens take time out to work abroad themselves. The number of recruitment agencies recruiting British-qualified nurses to work in these countries confirms that there is a buoyant exchange of capabilities going on and international migration consists of an in- and outflow of people and skills.

The following case study is that of a female migrant nurse from India. She is in her early thirties, married and was recently joined by her husband. Her story highlights the complexity of motivating factors that made her decide to come to work in Britain and then the subsequent frustration when she realised that she was stuck working in a care home under discriminatory conditions with little hope of rekindling her professional career.

> Actually my main reason to come over here is nice hospitals, so I said I can settle here. So I can work as a nurse here, so I can improve my knowledge and all these things. And also the other thing is the salary also, good salary.

I come through the agency. She (the manager of the recruitment agency) asked us to pay £2000, actually my friends all paid £2000 each. So after that she said, your work permit is quite costly or something like that, I don't know what is going on here. So you need to pay £2500. We have no contract because she assured the permit for four years and we got a visa for four years. But there is no contract. You need to work under this company for these many years.

I have a flat now with my husband. But my friends, they are paying £280, and some of them more than that for accommodation. That's why some of my friends are still waiting to bring their husbands. So as soon as our husbands come over to England we need to find other accommodation. If their husbands are working in the same home, then they are given accommodation there. They are not nurses. Some have done computer course, they are giving the nursing care. £5 per hour. 42 hours a week. Sometimes it's 8.00am to 2.00pm sometimes 2.00pm to 8.00pm. But most of the days I used to do 8.00am to 8.00pm, because you want to get as many hours as possible to earn £800 per month. I need to pay the rent and the phone. There are a lot of things, it is quite expensive. So I need to do some extra shift. I work most of the days. Sometimes 58–60 hours. No overtime payment. Nothing extra, nothing extra. British nurses they get £7.05 because now, the union came. All the local staff they get £7.05 each on weekends. So most of the nurses, I mean local nurse, they are working on Saturday and Sunday. They pay for us less, they need to pay £5.36, they do not pay us (migrant nurses) £7 something.

Life is too expensive. So that's why we need to work all hours and days. Some of the British staff they work as Care Assistants and some of them have no experience at all, they have worked in business or as a hairdresser or those kinds of different areas. So night time if they work they will get £8. But for us the same thing £5.36.

Actually in the home what we are doing is, in the morning we used to get the residents ready – I mean wash them and dress them. Then make them sit in the lounge. Then they need to get their breakfast. All the things we need to bring from the kitchen and serve the breakfast for all of them and clean the place and wash the plates and put it back again. Then again if inbetween they want to go to toilet or other things like that, we need to do that and take them to the toilet. And then we need to do the beds. Then we need to do the laundry. Then again sometimes we need to clean the toilet. Not sometimes, most of the times. I used to cry – you know – my friends as well. We need to clean the toilet you know! So terrible thing!

My mother tongue is Hindi. So I can speak Hindi. Then I was studying, so I can speak Tamil and I was in Malaysia so I can speak Malaysia language. I finished secondary school, left secondary school at age of 15. Then for two years I was in college. Then I was in college and then, I went for the lab vaccination course for one year. Then again after that I went for the nursing. I was working in India for four years then.

I try to get adaptation to be registered as a nurse in England. I wrote to nearly 50 hospitals, they replied, they said I am sorry, we are not running any adaptations. Some of the hospitals they said sorry we are giving places only to the candidates living in south London or north London or west London or central London. That's what they say. NMC letters says for me only need three months adaptation because I got experience, but the adaptation for some others is six months. I can not do adaptation in this care home, under the company.

I will go to work in hospital even if they are not running an adaptation, or if they are not recruiting candidates from India. If they start an adaptation, we would all be prepared to start adaptation next month, so those who want to come and join. But instead of that what they are doing? They will recruit the persons from India directly.

So still we are here, working in the care homes. Because nowadays the NHS all they are giving money for is the agencies, not nurses who are already in Britain. So the agencies will straight away go to the different country and they are recruiting the people from there. Everything is going through the agencies.

While this story make many of the issues faced by migrant nurses explicit, it needs to be noted that experiences in private care homes differ from those of nurses working in the NHS. While many NHS employers may not tap into the resources migrant nurses already living in the country have to offer, at least once they are being employed, they are generally treated more fairly and equally than they would be in the less well regulated private care sector. This is not to say that the private care sector does not have any regulatory framework – it has, however, its implementation is less stringently monitored.

Threats and persecution

Threats and persecution are the reasons why refugees decide to flee their countries of origin in search of a safer place to live. While some refugees clearly have a say in where they migrate to, many leave without knowing where they will end up. As was pointed out in the earlier chapters, many seek refuge in neighbouring countries in the hope that the situation in their homeland will stabilise sufficiently for them to return in due course, yet some will never be able to do so. In most cases forced migration, by definition, does not come about as a result of a planned, equal discussion among all members of the household. Other issues, such as available routes of flight and the need to leave urgently, may be overriding personal preferences and there is little time for sentiments.

The following experience highlights the suddenness and unexpectedness typical of refugee migration and the hurdles associated with accessing employment for migrant nurses belonging to this category. The following case study is taken from a 44-year-old female nurse who has two children and was separated from her husband. She had lived in the French-speaking Republic of Congo.

> The problem is I was not prepared to come to England, it was so quick. I didn't know any word in English. It was very difficult, I wanted to work as a nurse but I couldn't. I start by doing three-month English course. After that I went to UKCC [now NMC] to apply for registration, but it didn't work because I couldn't speak any English. I decided to go to a college and study health and science and I got accepted. I wanted to restart nursing training again and heard about a refugee organisation offering courses to prepare nurses for adaptation course. I applied and I did my interview and passed. Then I did three months pre-adaptation course. It helped me a lot to understand the system and then go for adaptation course. I went to Home Office, applied for a work permit and they gave it to me. I don't want to depend on social services: I have been independent in my country, I would like to be independent here.

Drawing on the description of the hurdles that refugee nurses need to go through, as outlined in Chapter 3, the fact that refugees do not generally plan their journey to Britain has implications for employment, as it can mean that:

- they may be traumatised and/or separated from their families, with no means of contacting family members
- they then face the scrutiny of the British immigration system, with all the uncertainties that this causes
- they can have no or little English language skills
- they may have left all professional documents and proof of qualifications and experience behind, with little opportunity of obtaining references
- they may have no or little knowledge about the employment process when they first arrive.

The procedures related to the immigration and employment processes do not convey the depth of personal experiences that individuals undergo and the level of uncertainty related to the outcome of the processes, particularly in cases of forced migration. A 28-year-old female nurse from Moldova made this explicit:

> For nurses from abroad, they see paper, but not the people. People have lots of difficulties to start. It is a very complicated process.

Immigrants and asylum seekers coming to Britain were formerly automatically allowed to apply for a work permit. This right has been replaced by a range of constrictions which aim to stop illegal employment.[14] Yet making it illegal for asylum seekers to work while their applications are being considered can force some to work without permission in the black market economy – an option not available for migrant nurses working in the NHS. The following comment made by a male migrant nurse in his twenties confirms this:

> There are a lot of people here from my country, they work in restaurants or they work illegally. But if you are a nurse, a doctor or something it is not possible to work illegally. In fact I save money here and my dream is to do further studies and once I have achieved it, and God willing I will achieve it and if they don't give me indefinite leave to remain I am happy to return. The status is making me feel unsettled, it will be a problem to me if they tell me to leave the country before I finish my studies. I am very grateful to them because they are allowing me to work. They have given me permission to work.

Until the Home Office has decided permanent residence status, the migrant nurse's continuation to work depends on the employer applying for work permits on behalf of the nurse and unfortunately not all employers are familiar with the processes and documentation involved. For example, the following 36-year-old female refugee nurse from Burundi was suspended from working for a week while the hospital tried to come to terms with her status:

> I have to explain to her that I don't have passport but just travel documents – 'Why don't you have passport?' You then have to explain, I am refugee, I have this and this document. She called the manager, and the manager called the ward manager and then all the people knew about my immigration status because of passing this to the sister and the sister called the nurse up, things like that. And I feel bad myself. I tried to explain to them, but the problem is that they didn't believe that I was telling them the truth. My papers are at the Home Office, I can't go to the Home Office, I can't push them. I don't have that power that I can go to the Home Office and tell them I need this and this. All I can do is talk to my lawyer and ask a letter to explain to you my situation in this country. Which I did and they refused the letter, they did not want it. They want a Home Office letter. Then my lawyer called me and she also called the hospital to explain to them – they still refused, but then she gave them the Home Office number. Once they rang, they were ashamed because I had explained everything.

Such uncertainties are extremely distressing and the nurse involved had contacted the author several times in tears and was extremely anxious about her future employment security and the hospital management's lack of understanding of her situation.

On the one hand employment can make an important positive contribution to refugees' self-worth and well-being. On the other hand the disclosure of personal information about the journey to Britain may not be something that many refugee nurses feel comfortable sharing at work. Nevertheless, the experience of distress, suffering, possibly war and flight from a dangerous country builds individuals' identity, which can affect motivation, and if responses to disclosure are positive, can lead to feelings of being 'respected'.

The following 41-year-old refugee nurse from Burundi not only shared some of these elements of her story with colleagues at work, but moreover expressed the link to work-related motivation, opposing any prejudices that refugees just come to 'beg or live off benefits'. With many refugees shying away from openly talking about the details of their immigration status, the following example is a rare exception:

> In the beginning they [colleagues, the hospital managers and doctors] were just asking questions, like laughing or something. I got the impression that they didn't understand what it was to be a refugee. Most of the people [in Britain], they think a refugee is someone who don't know [anything], or they are people who want to beg. But when I went to the hospital, I didn't want to hide anything. I wanted people to hear what that is to be a refugee. It's a situation that anyone, anywhere can get into ... they didn't know anything what was going on in the world. They have in their mind a refugee, who is someone who steals – so all the thieves are refugees. Because I told them about my story, everyone knew and everyone accepts that, and even the doctors came up and said: 'I didn't know you were one of the refugees'. She asked me many questions and that was really something. That brought it to the attention of so many people. Refugees are not just people who come here to beg. Refugees are not just people who come here to better their situation. They wanted to know: 'What is a refugee?' and 'How did you get from there to here and how did you come?'

She went on to express how the experience of sharing her story at work made her feel:

> It gives the refugee much respect, because you explain the situation and working with them they find, 'Oh a refugee is not someone who don't know [anything]. It is just a human being who can be able to do things for themselves.' ... Some of the refugees, they are very much motivated, especially that they have got the chance in this country which needs nurses.

Even when migrants are granted a work permit, such documents provide neither employment security nor do they settle the residence status of immigrants, and the following comment made by a 33-year-old female nurse from Romania indicated the dependency on employer's goodwill:

> If you come from India, for example, you need a work permit and then it expires and you need another work permit. They apply for that. Then you are not allowed to move and even if you want to move you need a reference from them. So you always need something.

Another example is that of a refugee nurse, who nine years after leaving Rwanda still had not received a permanent decision about her asylum claim from the Home Office. Contrary to her undecided immigration status, she had established herself professionally and had not only gained registration as a nurse in Britain, but had also been promoted to F-grade and was supervising colleagues on the ward, as well as supporting other migrant nurses during their integration process. As a result she felt more rooted in Britain, with nothing to go back to in Rwanda:

> I could not go back, I have nothing left there, where would I start? My kids are settled here.

She went on to outline how she had experienced the key difference between refugees' and other migrants' motivation for migration. She emphasised the point that, compared with other groups of migrants, refugees did not have many alternatives when deciding to flee:

> Sometimes it is hard to work, because staff they don't understand. They don't understand, even you have some overseas-trained nurses from Nigeria, from Ghana, but they only come here to look for a job. There are many reasons to come here. They wanted to work, but for us [as refugees] it is something different. You can't go back and leave ... you apply for your immigration status ... I always tell them: 'I flee my country. I didn't have any choice, I didn't have any choice.' We don't talk about that because they [other migrants] don't understand, they don't understand. Some people who just came here long time ago or their parents were here. They don't have the same experience. We want peace.

Her statement that refugee nurses did 'not have any choice' about coming to Britain and 'want peace' significantly affected how she perceived her integration at work. She saw employment as a key stepping-stone in rebuilding her life in an environment that provided stability and security.

Migrant nurses, regardless of their reasons for coming to another country, such as Britain, appreciate the opportunities to develop a professional career, earning a decent wage and extending their professional horizons, and most desire to maintain an existence independent of state support.

Motivations to work

Emotions experienced throughout employment can be a reliable indicator of job satisfaction and therefore relate to the *intrinsic motivation* of individuals to work. Migrant nurses, depending on their experiences of migration, report on the one hand positive work-related feelings, of confidence, respect, trust, security and self-worth, and on the other hand also negative feelings, such as isolation, despair, anxiety and fear, particularly during the early stages of their integration into a new employment context. Particularly during the early phase of their integration, many migrants in the empirical research stated that they experienced phases of severe gloominess, stress and despondency. These negative emotions contrasted with those experienced once registration as a nurse in Britain was achieved, which was accompanied by feelings of confidence and happiness.

While private feelings and personal expressions are apparently irrelevant for the formal part of the organisational role,[15] in practice they play an important role in organisational life.[16] Fisher *et al.*[17] emphasise that among other possible effects 'emotions at work' impact on effectiveness, satisfaction, commitment, well-being, stress and health.

Emotions form one aspect of individuals' needs and appear in Maslow's theory about the hierarchy of needs as feelings of self-esteem, confidence, achievement, independence, recognition and attention, with not all being of equal significance for all employees. In addition to these positive emotions, workers may also experience more negative feelings in relation to their work, such as stress, being distrusted, feeling bored or nervous. Therefore a range of emotions can be experienced in relation to work. Happiness is a positive feeling, expressing pleasure, contentment and satisfaction (Oxford Dictionary, 1974). Feelings of happiness can be related to a positive self-esteem and confidence, thus feeling 'in control' or 'empowered'.

Rowlands[18] points out that despite a lack of definition of *empowerment*, it relates to giving power to those who are marginalised, enabling them to participate in decision making. On a relational level, empowerment relates to the ability to negotiate and influence the nature of relationships and decisions made. Empowerment builds confidence and relates to the delegation of tasks and decision making to the most appropriate level of responsibility and includes low-ranking employees. *Trust* is crucial to the empowerment of individual employees and where employees are trusted to contribute their ideas and effort they are empowered. In contrast, if employees feel distrusted or disempowered they are in fear and less likely to make suggestions for improvement.[19]

Negative work-related feelings, such as *stress* or *gloom* can have a number of causes.[20] The individual may be overstretched and not have the ability to do the job, they may be discriminated against by fellow workers, they may perceive their pay as too low or praise and recognition could be absent. For example reported feelings of stress due to overload, tight deadlines or bad relationships with co-workers are increasingly common.[21,22] Stress derives from the Latin word *stringere*, meaning to draw tight. External forces are seen as exerting pressure upon the individual, leading to strain. Selye[23] described three stages of stress: first, an 'alarm reaction', the initial phase of lowered resistance; second, 'resistance' as a stage of maximum adaptation, hopefully with a successful return to equilibrium; however, if the stress agent continues, the individual can move to the third stage, which is 'exhaustion and collapse'. Aspects of the workplace or job role can be a considerable source of stress for individuals.[24]

There are individual and organisational symptoms of stress. The individual ones can include a depressed mood, feeling 'gloomy', excessive drinking, irritability and chest pain. The organisational symptoms include high absenteeism, labour turnover, difficult work relationships and a poor quality of performance.[25] The Oxford Dictionary describes 'gloom' as a feeling of sadness and helplessness and can be a negative outcome of stress. The number of days lost in Britain from work for certain mental and stress-related causes has been steadily increasing.

A distribution of feelings over a period of four weeks in the survey showed that personal factors also influence the way nurses felt about their work environment with some feeling more stressed and gloomy or more happy than others. When comparing emotions at work among different groups of nurses who responded to the survey, it became clear that age was also a decisive factor. Migrant nurses under the age of 32 years (chosen as a cut-off-point as it created almost equal sample sizes) reported lower levels of job satisfaction and higher levels of work-related stress than nurses who were older than 32 years. Explanations for these differences can only be tentative, but as age can correspond with employment tenure, migrant nurses at the beginning of their careers may experience day-to-day responsibilities as more stretching than older nurses who have been working for longer. This becomes an issue of concern among an ageing workforce and could be linked to high attrition rates, causing younger nurses not to stay in the profession.

Having skills and personal strengths and abilities recognised and affirmed by team members, supervisors and clients illustrates the intrinsic aspect of work-related motivation.

Extrinsic motivation, mostly referring to wage or salary, causes some people to work hard and put in considerable effort.[26,27] Yet there are obvious flaws with this notion, because most pay is not directly performance-related and individuals may reach their own performance peak irrespective of what they are paid. Extrinsic motivation becomes important, though, when employees are demotivated because they perceive themselves to be relatively underpaid compared to other categories of workers or when the buying power of their salary is insufficient for their perceived needs, and a number of migrant nurses referred to pay issues when questioned about their perception of working in Britain.

Below are examples of what migrant nurses had to say, reflecting mixed feelings about the level of pay compared to the effort put into work and the financial needs that nurses need to meet.

- 'There is too much pressure and too little payment, so you don't feel valued.'
- 'The salary is very low and not enough to support my family back in our country.'
- 'The pay is higher to what we get from our local jobs back in the Philippines, we find this better as far as financial matters are concerned.'

When asked what changes to their workplace they would like to see, they mentioned:

- improved salaries
- access to affordable housing or better staff accommodation
- access to childcare facilities.

The following comment sums up the dilemma of a migrant nurse who had been directly recruited from the Philippines to work in an NHS hospital:

> I left my three-bedroom house to come here to suffer like this – for what? The next thing I did was to go to the bank to ask for a mortgage. They offered me £90 000, which can buy one bedroom. That is useless for my family. Now the NHS Trust and government are introducing help for key workers. I applied and got the letter saying that because I am not a permanent resident in the UK I didn't qualify. I think it is total discrimination.

Some individuals perceive the exchange relationship between their input (in the form of shift work, working unsociable hours, stress and responsibility at work, working with too few permanent staff) as unfair compared to the outcome in terms of pay. In addition, the problems of living in inappropriate accommodation or worrying about relatives' well-being as a result of low pay negatively affects job satisfaction and in turn the amount of effort nurses are able to put into the job.

According to Parkinson,[28] the feelings that nurses express in relation to their employment can be a useful indicator of how they perceive their relationships with supervisors and colleagues to be and to what extent they are able to identify with facets of work and therefore commit to the organisation or workgroup. Work-related emotions can also be influenced by individual/personal factors, confirming the complex correlation between personal and work-related identities.

The themes of emotions and motivation reappear in the analyses of integration, relationships at work and contributions made by migrant nurses presented in the following chapters.

References

1 Shamir B (1996) Meaning, self and motivation in organizations. In: RM Steers, LW Porter and GA Bigley (ed) *Motivation and Leadership at Work* (6e). McGraw-Hill, London.

2 Adams JS (1965) Inequity in social exchange. In: L Berkowitz (ed) *Advances in Experimental Social Psychology, Vol. 2*. Academic Press, New York.

3 Maslow AH (1943) A theory of motivation. *Psychological Review*. **50**: 370–96.

4 Vroom VH (1964) *Work and Motivation*. Wiley, New York.

5 Porter LW and Lawler EE III. (1968) *Managerial Attitudes and Performance*. Richard D. Irwin Inc., Homewood.

6 Huczynski A and Buchanan D (2001) *Organizational Behaviour: an introductory text* (4e). Prentice Hall International, London.

7 Staw BM (1976) *Intrinsic and Extrinsic Motivation*. General Learning Press, Morristown, NJ.

8 Nussbaum M (2000) *Women and Human Development: the capabilities approach*. Cambridge University Press, Cambridge.

9 NMC (2004) www.nmc-uk.org/nmc/main/advice/enrolledNursing.html (accessed 2005).

10 BBC News (1998) Luring nurses back into the NHS. 23 September 1998. http://news.bbc.co.uk/1/hi/health/178226.stm.

11 Seccombe I, Smith G, Buchan J *et al.* (1997) *Enrolled Nurses: a study for the UKCC*. IES Report 344. Institute of Employment Studies, Brighton.

12 McKay S and Winkelmann-Gleed A (2005) *Migrant Workers in the East of England: final research report*. WLRI, London Metropolitan University and EEDA, London and Cambridge.

13 Sriskandarajah D Cooley L and Reed H (2005) *Paying Their Way: the fiscal contribution of immigrants in the UK*. ippr, London.

14 Home Office. (2004) Working in the UK. Work permit arrangements. 20 February 2004. www.workingintheuk.gov.uk/working_in_the_uk/en/homepage/work_permits/overview_of_process/people_who_do_not.html? Home Office, London.

15 Fineman S (1993) *Emotion in Organizations*. Sage, London.

16 Brown RB (1997) Emotion in organizations, the case of British university business school academics. *Journal of Applied Behavioural Science*. **33**(2): 247–62.

17 Fisher CD and Ashkanasy NM 2000. The emerging role of emotions in work life: an introduction. *Journal of Organizational Behaviour*. **21**(2): 123–9.

18 Rowlands J (1997) *Questioning Empowerment*. Oxfam, Oxford.

19 Mullins LJ (2002) Managerial behaviour and effectiveness. In: LJ Mullins (ed) *Management and Organisational Behaviour* (6e). Prentice Hall, London.

20 Cooper CL and Payne R (1990) *Causes, Coping, and Consequences of Stress at Work*. Wiley, Chichester.

21 Crouch D (2003) Combating Stress. *Nursing Times*. **99**(5): 22–5, 4 February.

22 Rana E and Roberts Z (2003) Stress standards warning. *People Management*. **23 January**: 7.

23 Selye H (1946) *Stress Without Disaster*. J.B. Lippincott, Philadelphia.

24 Elkin AJ and Rosch PJ (1990) Promoting mental health at the workplace: the prevention side of stress management. *Occupational Medicine: State of the Art Review*. **5**(4): 739–54.

25 Arnold J, Cooper CL and Robertson IT (1998) *Work Psychology*. Financial Times Publishing, London.

26 Locke EA and Latham GP (1990) *A Theory of Goal Setting and Task Performance*. Prentice Hall, Englewood Cliffs.

27 Locke EA and Latham GP (1996) Goal Setting Theory: an introduction. In: RM Steers, LW Porter and GA Bigley (eds) *Motivation and Leadership at Work* (6e). McGraw Hill, New York.

28 Parkinson B (1995) *Ideas and Realities of Emotion*. Routledge, London.

CHAPTER 5

Integrating: linking motivation and relationships

Relationships at work, namely interactions with colleagues of varying professional levels, mentors and supervisors, form key points of contact which can enable or impede newcomers from identifying with aspects of their new working environment. Individual experiences of such relationships can be encouraging or discouraging and such encounters are linked to work-related motivation as they affect the individuals' well-being at work.

Facets of the employment context, such as 'motivation', 'relationships at work' and self-reported feelings or 'emotions at work' mitigate the integration of all workers, but particularly Black and minority ethnic workers, into work and subsequently into an important part of society.[1–5] There are two fundamentally different approaches to integration: first, that of conformity, of cultural assimilation which believes in a common national culture with collective values, ideals, moral beliefs and social practices, and second, that of genuinely viewing cultural and other human difference and variety as enriching.[6]

In line with Parekh's view on multiculturalism, the author's views are based on appreciating diversity as a positive contribution to society and within that to the organisations employing a varied workforce. The following plea made by a male refugee nurse reflects this two-way process as a basis for integration:

> I just want them to respect me, I have respect of British people.

However, for all colleagues to truly respect the 'other' requires careful management of relationships and also a well thought-out approach in which tasks are being performed.

It is in the expression of interactions with colleagues and supervisors that internationally qualified nurses experience the motivational aspects of their work which can foster or hinder their commitment to the work-group and wider organisation. Concepts of social identity theory, organisational commitment and motivation theories taken from the organisational behaviour and psychology literature can therefore aid the process of understanding some of the underlying dynamics and help to place individual encounters into a wider context. In addition, writings from anthropology provide further understanding of personal identity issues related to international migration. Identity issues create opportunities to overcome the barriers between indigenous and internationally trained individuals, and 'them' and 'us' thinking. Such insights can help to better understand nurses' experiences and inform recommendations related to their integration.

The literature on social identity[7–9] explains that individuals naturally form relationships with those who appear similar to them. Tajfel *et al.*[10] explain that such similarities are based on superficial, observable characteristics, such as age, gender, dress code or ethnicity. Hogg[7] *et al.* go on to say that self-identification is closely linked to identification with a wider social group as individuals seek a positive social identity by belonging to an in-group, thus enhancing their self-worth. Individuals who are prevented from socially identifying at their workplace might remain or become 'a stranger', someone who feels isolated and socially excluded. Social exclusion looks at 'the process through which individuals or groups are wholly or partially excluded from full participation in the society in which they live'.[11] Understanding and managing the facets related to work-related identities and motivators can only benefit the integration of migrants. Moreover, they can be a precursor to their contribution to capacity within the organisation.

Relationships with colleagues, mentors and supervisors form part of the informal aspect of organisational life, presenting a window through which individuals view and experience their work environment. With most people spending a substantial part of their daily lives at work, interactions with colleagues impinge not only on work-related, but also on personal issues as relationships develop into friendships among colleagues. Therefore dealings with supervisors and colleagues can greatly affect the way individuals feel about their work,[12] and commitment to the workgroup is important, as this is where employees communicate most closely with each other, get to know each other and express loyalty, as well as work out conflict.[13] It is acknowledged that poor relationships at work are reflected in low levels of interest and trust among employees, leading to a lack of support and low levels of job satisfaction, motivation and well-being at work.[14] Thus interacting with people can either be a source of encouragement or stress. Moreover, feelings of either achievement and confidence or stress and failure not only influence the individuals' integration into work, but also their self-identity. Related to their loss of previously held status,[15] migrants may feel more vulnerable to negative aspects of work relationships than indigenous employees would. Consequently, particularly for migrants who are new to work in Britain, the experiences of relationships at work can be an important factor in encouraging or hindering their integration at the workplace and ultimately in society.

Another important feeling reflected in relationships among a diverse workforce is that of *fairness*, which relates to Equity Theory, *see* p. 42. Fairness and equality are also understood through the concepts of distributive and procedural justice. Distributive justice comes into play when employees are not satisfied with rewards and outcomes in response to their efforts. Procedural justice is reflected in the behaviour of colleagues and supervisors relating to interactive justice, which is concerned with the fairness of the process itself.[16,17] Fairness and procedural justice as well as emotions at work offer an individual picture of job satisfaction related to day-to-day work.

Relationships with 'others' at work

This section presents examples of individual encounters experienced by migrant nurses, starting with relationships with colleagues, before going on to relationships with mentors and finally supervisors and other managers. The comments made by migrant nurses about these relationships question some of the labels used to define people groups and highlight nuances in these relationships. British-trained nurses and indeed other professional groups may attribute a similar weight to relationships at work. However, as the migrant nurses are undergoing an adaptation programme which can be more or less structured and take place in a cohort or just a small group of other internationally qualified nurses, they can often feel more isolated and insecure. Within this context relationships can have far-reaching consequences on workplace integration.

The migrant nurse's colleagues can be fully or partially trained, some are temporary staff, such as agency nurses and bank nurses, with others working full-time with a permanent contract. They are British or potentially also internationally qualified nurses working in various specialities, grades and levels of responsibilities and they form part of the close workgroup that migrants, as newcomers, join.

Relationships with colleagues

The following experience shows that attitudes of colleagues can greatly ease integration. Being kind and helpful towards migrants by understanding that procedures may be different in other countries and by explaining equipment and British nursing procedures expresses acceptance and support towards the newcomers. The following 44-year-old nurse from the Congo had experienced such colleagues and this is what she said:

> The permanent staff they are very, very helpful, when they did a special care procedure for a patient, they call me in to show me what to do. Everything, the equipment, they tell me how to do things. It depends on the person,

because some of them, they are kind, understand that I come from another country where things are different.

Other migrant nurses point out that the initiative to ask for help also lies with them, as they have a responsibility to find out how to put procedures into practice and which protocols to follow. Migrant nurses are not necessarily less experienced, but have gained their experience in sometimes very different work settings. Yet colleagues have to present themselves as approachable in order for the newcomer to be brave enough to seek help without being made to feel inferior. This can be done by being open to also asking the migrants about their past nursing experience in order to learn how things are done elsewhere and to show the respect called for.

The following comment made by a male nurse from the Middle East highlights how personal issues can overlap with work-related ones as he talked to his colleagues about non-work-related concerns:

> My colleagues are helping me as much as they can. They are all acting in a very professional way. I think they are glad to help me and they are not only helping me in professional things – sometimes, in the break, we talk about other things: if they have problems or if I have problems. They are trying to help as much as they can. They have a different cultural background compared to me, we are from different countries and we are different. You can act in two ways: one is just to do your job and not get involved other than the professional, other than the nursing. Don't talk about anything else and don't go out with them. The other way is that you can talk to them about some personal things and share as much as you can in a social event. If you choose that way you will not be so isolated. It is true that you will have some cultural clashes at some times though.

In the empirical study few problems were reported about migrant nurses' relationships with fully qualified nursing colleagues, instead they were found to be *helpful, supportive, encouraging* and *approachable*. Internationally qualified nurses' interactions with colleagues who were not registered as fully qualified nurses presented a different picture and often relationships with auxiliary nurses, Health Care Assistants and agency nurses were experienced by the migrant nurses as problematic. The shortage of fully qualified nursing staff means that many newcomers depend on the support given by lesser-trained colleagues while learning about nursing procedures in Britain. There are doubtless many auxiliaries or agency nurses who are hard-working and supportive of their colleagues and at the same time there are fully qualified nurses who are unsupportive and prejudiced. Yet on the whole it appears more likely that lesser qualified nurses and those on temporary working arrangements may view migrant nurses as a threat to their own employment security and may therefore resent them. It is this that reflected in some of the experiences migrants reported when interacting with them. A 41-year-old nurse from Burundi gave an example of an auxiliary nurse who felt threatened and, even though an isolated incident, it makes the underlying issues explicit:

> All the opposition was from the auxiliary nurses and the agency nurses. They made it clear and said: 'You take our job, if you come and if you start work here at this hospital.' And I said: 'Well, you could take a permanent job too.' But they didn't like that, they don't want that, they just want money, more money. The auxiliaries walked out and left me without help. So they made it very difficult for me. They could write something down, to show that I have made mistakes. They did that and showed it to the ward manager and he said: 'Well, she is just learning.' There is something going on, maybe I was checking drugs with another nurse and they wrote something else down. I said: 'I do make mistakes, but not when I am checking with a second nurse, when it is two of us checking.' That nurse had a few problems at the hospital.

Even though some auxiliary nurses or nurses on temporary or agency contracts may perceive that migrant nurses working full-time put their jobs under threat, there is no evidence to indicate that any have actually lost their jobs. On the contrary, in nursing alone there are nationally in Britain 3.1% of posts currently unfilled. Yet other migrant nurses also reported similar experiences with their lesser-qualified colleagues or those on temporary working arrangements:

> It is the healthcare workers, they want to be boss and they speak their own language when they gather together in front of the patient.

> Those from the agency, they are not approachable.

Such interpersonal issues can undermine team dynamics and impact on the effectiveness with which the workgroup operates.

In addition to the professional and employment grades that colleagues hold, the role of language and cross-cultural communication are important factors influencing relationships with colleagues, which are based on verbal and non-verbal forms of communication. The following examples highlight stumbling blocks related to migrants' *verbal communication skills*. A lack of ability in speaking English, despite having successfully passed the required English language tests, can undermine migrants' self-confidence. The following 29-year-old nurse from the Philippines noted the following when comparing the British-trained nurses' interaction with doctors to her own:

> There is a big difference, those who were trained in Britain, they are so confident with the things and have confidence with communication, with talking

to the doctor, colleagues, even patients. But those internationally trained nurses . . . you know, there are communication barriers, they are big.

When English is acquired as a second or third language, difficulties in everyday comprehension can cause difficulties with comprehending slang or humour, which is culture-bound. Sarcasm or irony, common elements of British humour, are often puzzling for migrants as they do not translate very well and they can be offensive to individuals.

Migrants' perceptions of their colleagues' reactions to their non-native English accents also seems to affect relationships. Not feeling understood despite trying one's best to speak another language creates boundaries to integration into the existing work team. The following example, given by a 36-year-old nurse from Burundi, highlights this:

> At first I was going to run because I will never speak English like an English-speaker. My pronunciation, my accent will not change. Some people, they say: 'What is this?' – are you with me? They look at each other. Sometimes you feel really bad. They turn to the other person: 'Did you hear what she said?' Some are very young, I am not sure if all of them are English, but all of them they speak English. They didn't complain, but they just took off my name from the rota.

Others believe that because of the lack of language skills colleagues assume that they are not well enough educated or did not attend proper schools. This relates to a general ignorance of other countries and cultures, many of which may be perceived as 'primitive' and 'less developed'. Instead of recognising that ignorance can lead to narrow-mindedness and being open to learn from others who have lived elsewhere, some conceal their fear of acknowledging their own lack of knowledge by responding with prejudice.

Cross-cultural communication is very complex and the use of language in particular can build up or damage relationships at work and thus make integration a problematic process. Generally, though, nurses seem to like working in teams and are aware of the importance of getting along with each other, as the following comments in response to the question 'What do you enjoy most about your job?' indicate:

> Working with a very co-operative team reduces stress at work.

> Teamwork makes the job more comfortable.

> Team working encourages commonalities, despite hard work, and promotes harmony and quality.

The importance of team working was also confirmed in responses given to the question: 'What do you enjoy least about your job?':

Working with an unco-operative team increases stress.

Working with nurses with no dedication to serve, they are destroying the essence of nursing.

Nurses who think they are perfect.

The relationships between migrant nurses and their colleagues reflect different facets of the journey towards integration and show some of the complexities between work-related and personal issues, such as attitudes towards strangers, understanding of different cultures and willingness to support members of the work team who seem weaker.

On the whole most nurses in the empirical study rated the support they received from colleagues as quite high, but the 114 female nurses in the survey sample rated the support they received both from colleagues and from supervisors as significantly higher than the male respondents. Explanations for this can only be hypothetical, for example one could say that women are generally more relationship-oriented and therefore rate them higher than men, who may be more focused on other aspects of their working lives. On the other hand, men may have higher expectations of the relationships with supervisors or colleagues when coming to the UK and may be more disappointed than the women.

Relationships with mentors

Migrant nurses are often very experienced professionals, as well as mature individuals, who then have to start again at the bottom of the career ladder in Britain. This can be daunting, not only for them but also for those working closely with them. In the early phases of their employment, during their 'supervision/adaptation period', the most important relationship which is also key to the success of their registration as a nurse in Britain is their relationship with the assigned mentor. Anecdotal evidence from key informants in the NHS shows an equal amount of praise and criticism about the support migrants receive from their mentors.

Starting with the negative comments made by migrant nurses about their mentors, these often reflect the migrants' feelings of uncertainty, unmet expectations and of having lost familiar points of reference in their profession. A female nurse from Rwanda who is in her late forties made this comment:

Everything you know is different. I felt a bit strange, as they didn't know me. So, it's like they are not sure and it was a bit hard to integrate in the beginning.

Repeatedly migrant nurses seem to observe that their mentors often fail to remember their own beginnings as nurses and have probably never worked in an unknown, foreign environment. The same respondent commented on this by saying:

> They didn't remember how it was when they first started a job – in the first week, the first year, you know. Remember, we are not student nurses. I am not a student nurse. I am qualified. I have 25 years' experience of being a nurse. I have not started here, I am just adapting my knowledge.

A 33-year-old midwife from Iran described an extremely unsupportive relationship with her mentor which reduced her to tears and despair throughout large parts of her supervision period:

> My mentor, my supervisor, her behaviour and her attitude, honestly, at that point I just cried, just started to cry, I don't know – is there any regulation for those people? ... if I could get more encouragement, I wouldn't suffer from the impact or psychological. But with the behaviour of that mentor ... oh my God, nobody can believe it. My mentor is so discouraging, it is very hard.

She went on and expressed her helplessness:

> I don't know what to do, to go and complain or just to be treated like I was stupid, just because I have come from different area, different country.

It seems difficult to truly prepare mentors for their role, as so many aspects of interacting with a newcomer are based on individual personality rather than knowledge, and some may become more aware of the issues that matter to migrant nurses as time goes by and as they keep interacting with foreigners on a daily basis.

At the same time, the task of assessing a migrant nurse's abilities and competencies for being able to operate in the British healthcare system has to be taken seriously. This is where mentors have to be professional, distinguishing between personal, interpersonal and competency issues.

There are very practical aspects to the relationship between mentors and migrants which can lead to a successful or unsuccessful integration, such as:

- the fact that mentors need to be selected on their willingness to interact with migrants, not be forced into it on the basis of their status in the organisation
- the amount of time spent together
- the amount of face-to-face contact
- the amount of other responsibilities mentors carry reflects on the seriousness that is placed on their relationship with migrants
- the way in which the whole supervision/adaptation programme is organised

- the way in which mentors are prepared to be aware of some of the basic, universal cross-cultural issues
- the way in which personality clashes are addressed.

While feeling insecure in the new working environment, migrants really depend on positive encouragement from their mentors, as well as their practical help and support. The importance of this mentor–migrant relationship also becomes clear in the comment made by a male nurse in his twenties who appreciated the support and above all the respect he was given:

> She is as professional as possible, really good in a very professional way. She is very experienced. Sometimes, some nurses are unlucky, very unlucky with their mentor. I think I am very lucky with my mentor, she is respecting me.

Thus support can be exercised through a general attitude of valuing the 'other' and showing helpfulness through specific acts in specific circumstances, such as:

- going out of the way to photocopy some literature relevant to the nurse's success during the integration period
- positive introductions of the newcomer to the existing staff team, thus making their integration into the existing work team easier
- the passing on of relevant articles in nursing magazines
- trying to understand the migrant's background and level of knowledge and personal, as well as professional experience they hold
- being motivated about mentoring someone and seeing that person succeed.

The significance of the relationship between the newcomer and their mentors is unique and not only forms a stepping-stone towards integration, but also forms the basis of professional skills assessment, either facilitating or hindering the migrants' success in a different working environment. Moreover, because of the relative intimacy of the relationship, mentors can get to know the individual migrant more closely and thus build bridges between them and other members of staff and ultimately the wider organisation. At the same time, if this relationship deteriorates or breaks down, there can be far-reaching consequences not only for the nurse's professional registration and integration but also for his or her wider well-being.

Relationships with other supervisors and managers

Equally important to the mentors' relationship is the migrant nurse's relationship with other supervisors, such as ward sisters or ward managers. In fact, in some cases where the relationship with the mentor is not functioning very well, other supervisors are known to take on a 'mentoring role'.

Regardless of their relationship with the individual mentor, who is only spending a limited amount of time with the migrant nurse, the relationship with other supervisors who are a more constant feature in their day-to-day working lives is very important and characteristics of this relationship functioning well are:

- being generally supportive
- taking time to explain day-to-day routines
- encouraging the newcomer in taking up new responsibilities while supervising them
- offering themselves as a resource that is approachable, nurturing trust and confidence among the newcomers
- making the migrant feel confident by empowering them into doing new tasks
- being approachable and delegating responsibility to the migrant without overloading them, thereby displaying trust in the migrants' abilities
- recognising and affirming migrants' skills.

Affirmation of skills can go beyond the professional background, as some migrants have lived through stressful events in the past that were unique to their cultural background or migration experiences. This could make them either ideal or also very bad candidates for dealing with stressful situations at work. For example, a nurse from Kosovo was reported to have a calming influence on her team when the workload got stressful. Her experience of civil war had made her resilient in some situations that others perceived as stressful and her confidence in the team's ability to cope was also an encouragement for her colleagues and a stimulating challenge for herself. Her manager recognised and appreciated this as a strength:

> When things on the ward got stressful, she would say: 'this is not a major crisis, let's get on with it' and she would be a calming influence on the other nurses as a role model.

To be given such recognition by managers can truly enhance self-worth and confidence. Such motivation can also lead to high levels of job satisfaction and other positive work-related emotions. Other examples of managers' practical support include recognising personal responsibilities which impinge on individuals' work-related responsibilities, such as being the main carer for children or elderly relatives or having to sort out domestic issues which require visiting offices during certain times. The allocation of suitable shifts is not an issue exclusive to migrants. However, with many of them being separated from their normal support networks, they may take some time to re-establish themselves in a new living environment in addition to getting used to work. Other examples of support include the following:

- being sensitive to migrants' personal and family-related commitments and considering these when developing off-duty rotas
- ensuring that newcomers and existing members of staff are treated equally without favouritism towards the British-trained staff
- ensuring implementation of equal opportunities policies and procedures and advising newcomers where to seek help if they feel discriminated against
- developing interpersonal skills which reflect sensitivity for cultural and personal issues that individuals may have
- being professional and proficient in the support that is provided – this involves the supervisors being up-to-date on personnel management issues as well as on clinical ones
- being able to learn about others' cultural background and the way things are done differently without prejudging
- taking some time to get to know the newcomer a little and showing interest in their integration at work, asking how they are getting along – this can be very difficult: with many demands on managers and supervisors, the time spent on interpersonal issues can often fall short of the ideal.

Yet as the success of professional relationships also depends on interpersonal issues and individual personalities and to a lesser amount on the status individuals have in the organisational hierarchy, some of the successes or failures of relationships are symptomatic of that. Newcomers should know that failed relationships with colleagues or with some managers are not necessarily their fault and the organisational management should ensure that individuals' attitudes towards migrants do not impinge on their professional success. A 33-year-old nurse from Sierra Leone made this more explicit:

> For example a patient at A&E who needed transfer and I observed a nurse from the Philippines where the patient found it difficult to believe that she was in charge because she is from the Philippines. It will be difficult to change because some of the ward sisters, the way they treat you it is just their attitude. The management has nothing to do with that because they have grown up with that. Even when I am in class you can see that all the Black sit in one area and all the White in another – you feel so bad – even in a group of three or four the White just come and sit with the Whites. The lecturers try to change that, but it is very difficult. People just accept that it is like that because you can't change them.

Many migrants are determined in trying to make the most of given opportunities. Supportive interactions with colleagues, mentors and supervisors are a key element in succeeding in a new workplace, particularly when the integration process is partially managed through a one-to-one mentoring system. Interpersonal contacts at work impact on personal as well as work-related identities either positively or negatively. Relationships at work can therefore either be experienced as stimulating, encouraging and motivating or as stressful, demoralising and dispiriting. If the latter occurs, the effect of relationships can undermine feelings of confidence and self-esteem. Even though this applies to work-related relationships in general, regardless of ethnicity, gender or country of origin, newcomers appear particularly sensitive, as they have lost familiar relationships and points of identity. Relationships with mentors and supervisors are a central dimension of personal and work-related identity, motivation and integration, and even though relationships with supervisors might not necessarily affect commitment to peers in the workgroup, they may influence commitment to the profession, organisation and career.

References

1 Guest D, Peccei R and Thomas A (1993) The impact of employee involvement on organisational commitment and 'them and us' attitudes. *Industrial Relations Journal.* **24**(3): 191–201.

2 Coleman DF, Irving GP and Cooper CL (1999) Another look at the locus of control-organisational commitment relationship: it depends on the form of commitment. *Journal of Organizational Behavior.* **20**: 995–1001.

3 Clugston M (2000) The mediating effects of multidimensional commitment on job satisfaction and intent to leave. *Journal of Organisational Behaviour.* **21**: 477–86.

4 Tsui AS and O'Reilly CA (1989) Beyond simple demographic effects: the importance of relational demographic in superior-subordinate dyads. *Academy of Management Journal.* **32**(2): 402–23.

5 Wallace JE (1993) Professional and organisational commitment: Compatible or incompatible? *Journal of Vocational Behavior.* **42**: 333–49.

6 Parekh B (2000) *Rethinking Multiculturalism: cultural diversity and political theory.* Macmillan Press, London.

7 Hogg MA and Terry DJ (2000) Social identity and self-categorization processes in organizational contexts. *Academy of Management Review.* **25**(1): 121–40.

8 Harrison DA, Price KH and Bell MP (1998) Beyond relational demography: time and the effects of surface- and deep- level diversity on work group cohesion. *Academy of Management Journal.* **41**(1): 96–107.

9 Chatman JA, Polzer JT, Barsade SG *et al.* (1998) Being different yet feeling similar: the influence of demographic composition and organisational culture on work processes and outcomes. *Administrative Science Quarterly.* **43**: 749–80.

10 Tajfel H and Turner JC (1979) Social groups and identities. In: WP Robinson (ed) *Developing the Legacy of Henry Tajfel.* Butterworth-Heinemann, Oxford.

11 European Foundation (1995) *Public Welfare Services and Social Exclusion: the development of consumer-oriented initiatives in the European Union.* European Foundation for the Improvement of Living and Working Conditions, Dublin.

12 Makin P, Cooper CL and Cox C (1996) *Organizations and the Psychological Contract.* British Psychological Society, Leicester.

13 Kramer RM (1993) Cooperation and organisational identification In: JK Murnighan (ed) *Social Psychology in organisations: advances in theory and research.* Prentice Hall, Englewood Cliffs, New York.

14 Arnold J, Cooper CL and Robertson IT (1998) *Work Psychology.* Financial Times Publishing, London.

15 Haddad E (2002) The refugee: forging national identities. *Studies in Ethnicity and Nationalism.* **2**(2): 23–38.

16 Folger R (1987) In: RM Steers, LW Porter and GA Bigley (eds) *Motivation and Leadership at Work* (6e). McGraw-Hill, Singapore.

17 Cropanzano R and Folger R (1989) Referent Cognitions and Task Decision Autonomy: beyond equity theory. *Journal of Applied Psychology.* **74**(2): 293–9.

CHAPTER 6

Integrating: aspects of meeting the 'other'

The notion of 'otherness' is being constructed not by reflecting upon oneself, but by presuming characteristics of others. In addition to the relationships with colleagues, mentors and other supervisors or managers, there are further facets that signify the journey towards integration. When meeting 'strangers' we learn about ourselves and about the 'other' and different points of view or ways in which things are accomplished. This chapter therefore looks at language, culture and gender as expressions of the 'other' and examines migrant nurses' integration within this context.

> In Africa there is no stress working in hospitals, but you get to know more clinical procedures, you are forced to practice more. Here nurses work under stress, they work in fear of making mistakes and being held accountable, back home nurses are very respected.

Migrant nurses from regions such as the Middle East may have worked in relatively successful healthcare systems, while others from countries such as Ghana may even have worked in a healthcare system that was originally modelled on the British one. Thus some international approaches to nursing resemble the British nursing ethic more than others because of their shared colonial history.

Attitudes of prejudice among people are most commonly based on external characteristics, such as skin colour, texture of hair or accents, and even though 'ethnic labelling' has its shortcomings by stereotyping individuals and grouping them together, ethnic categories are part of ethnic monitoring in many organisations. While ethnic monitoring questions group individuals into categories such as 'White', 'Mixed', 'Asian', 'Black' or 'Chinese', with several sub-categories to each, this terminology is often not used when people describe themselves to others. For example, a migrant nurse may describe their own identity by stating that they are a 'refugee', a 'Palestinian', a 'woman' and 'mother'. Other self-definitions can include labels like: 'student', being

'African', 'Burundian', an 'Arab' or 'Rwandan', or they point to religious beliefs stating that as a 'Christian' they had suffered persecution in a Muslim country or as a 'Muslim' they feel awkward wearing a nurse's uniform in Britain and working with patients of a different gender to themselves. Therefore such self-definitions can differ greatly from how others, who only notice obvious appearances, perceive 'the stranger' within the work context.

One male migrant nurse encountered the following remarks, first from a patient and then from a colleague:

I don't want to be treated by a terrorist. [remark made by a patient]

and

All Arabs treat women like slaves. [remark made by a colleague to the same nurse]

It seems difficult to discern if any such clichés made to describe 'the stranger' are the result of ignorance and thoughtlessness or of prejudices. Moreover, universal statements about 'others' are made by British-trained nurses, as well as some internationally qualified nurses about other sub-groups of migrants.

Perceptions about the 'other' vary greatly and the following two examples indicate the extreme views expressed by two migrant nurses about the way they perceived their British-trained colleagues:

I think that British nurses are more organised than Pakistani nurses.

The average British nurse is not ready to work, so they always need support and if the support is not coming, they get hysterical.

Both statements are generalisations based on individual perceptions of working for a relatively brief period of less than a year with a finite number of British-trained nurses. Yet we all find ourselves thinking or expressing universal observations about other people around us, even though we neither know them properly nor fully understand if they are representative.

Consequently labels such as 'British', 'Pakistani', 'Jew' or 'Arab' are commonly used in order to describe people's behaviours, not just their geographical origins. For this they do not appear to be very useful categories, as individual encounters with 'others' vary and interpersonal encounters reveal commonalities as well as differences. The following comment provides an illustration of such commonalities among differently labelled groups of nurses.

A 95-year-old Jewish refugee doctor who had migrated from Germany to Britain during the 1930s mentioned the preference that British nurses who held Seventh Day Adventist beliefs had for working at the London Jewish Hospital. Working in a Jewish organisation enabled them to regularly celebrate the Sabbath, which would have been more difficult in other British hospitals:

About half of the nurses (at the London Jewish Hospital in the 1930s and 40s) were German Jewish, a third of them were Irish and very few were English. Most of these English ones were Seventh Day Adventists. Saturday was a holy day for them, they didn't need to do anything that was not urgent – there were no routine operations.

Differences in skin colour are a further, often more explicit, example of diversity than held religious beliefs and conclusions are readily drawn on the basis of someone 'looking' similar or different. As was made clear in the quote about skin colour and classroom behaviour above, conclusions and assumptions made on the basis of such surface-level diversity can lead to behaviour of inclusion or exclusion towards others.

True equality relates to procedural or interactive justice which is concerned with the fairness of the employment process reflected in the day-to-day behaviour of supervisors and colleagues. The survey conducted in the empirical study showed that most respondents perceived organisational procedures and equal opportunities policies as fairly implemented (mean of 4.22). However, this should not serve to neglect the few who have experienced serious discrimination as demonstrated in the distribution of survey respondents' perceptions of procedural fairness on a scale of 1 to 7, with a score of 7 being 'very fair', shown in Figure 6.1.

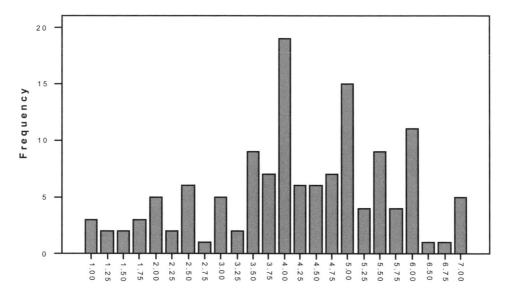

Figure 6.1   Procedural fairness – perceptions given by survey respondents.
Std. dev = 1.43; Mean = 4.22; N = 135.00.

The next figure, Figure 6.2 illustrates the distribution of responses related to perceptions of the implementation of equal opportunities policies, reflecting that most rated this as medium to high, with a score of 7 being the highest (mean of 4.76):

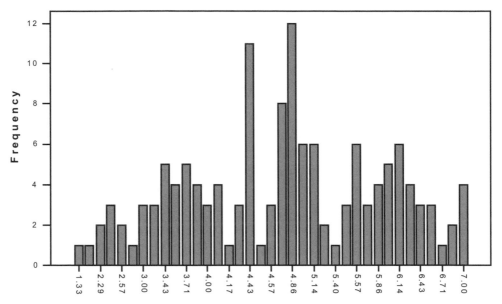

Figure 6.2   Equal opportunities – responses.
Std. Dev = 1.22; Mean = 4.76; N = 139.00.

Equality and procedural fairness reflects in the following work-related behaviours:

- implementing open communication procedures among all members of staff
- showing respect for migrant nurses and those who appear 'different', regardless of the nature of these differences (age, gender, ethnicity, disability)
- avoiding any form of discrimination
- truly adhering to the spirit of equal opportunities policies
- becoming credible and accountable in the way existing policies are implemented
- stopping incidences of bullying and harassing
- providing support to staff who feel discriminated against and helping them to utilise procedures to make themselves heard
- implementing flexible working hours to allow individuals space for personal commitments

The following examines issues such as language, racist attitudes and gender norms as symptoms of procedural inequality when engaging with the 'other'.

Meeting others – language

The use of language is a further expression of inclusion as well as exclusion. Language illustrates barriers between ethnically diverse groups of people, as it illustrates the creation of divisions and coalitions among individuals who are from different ethnic or racial backgrounds.

The following is an account between a migrant nurse from Burundi and her colleague from the Caribbean. On hearing that the Burundian nurse was fully qualified, but had trained in a different language, a personal encounter took place which contributed to a deeper understanding between 'strangers':

> There are nurses from Jamaica and they are from English-speaking countries. 'How long did you do your training?' one of these nurses asked me and I replied, 'Well, I did my training for four years' – and she looked at me in a very astonished way, saying: 'Is it true?' I said, 'Yes, but I didn't do my training in English, I did it in French.' – 'Oh really?'

The same nurse then went on to talk about her own experiences of feeling excluded while some sub-groups of internationally qualified nurses share a common language, providing them with a collective identity:

> Sometimes, I feel lonely, like I am on my own. No one is covering for me because when other groups of nurses from the Caribbean or Nigeria are together, it's like they are covering each other. If one of them does something, no one will make a big deal. But if you are on your own, no one is there for you and it is a bit difficult. It can't be very easy for them as well, but there is the language and they have so much in common.

Another phenomenon of shared language is that some migrant nurses may use their mother tongue when speaking to colleagues from the same ethnic background, which can equally be the case among colleagues from Europe and the Philippines, as well as other countries. With English being the shared language within the UK employment context, speaking in a language that is not understood by the majority can make colleagues and clients feel isolated, as this female nurse from the Philippines expressed:

> Some of the African nurses speak their own language. They also do this when they gather together in front of the patient. So, if you don't know the language you may think they are speaking about you.

Being excluded on the basis of language not only makes people feel isolated, but for newcomers it can enforce feelings of insecurity and 'not-belonging' in a place. The recognition of employees supporting each other on the basis of shared ethnic identity can exacerbate isolation of the minorities and hinder integration for those who are not part of that group. Thus the use of language creates boundaries, as it differentiates British-trained nurses, but also creates sub-groups of migrant nurses based on their native language. Language therefore defines parameters for social inclusion or exclusion and leads to individuals feeling accepted or isolated.

Meeting others: facets of racist attitudes

The Parekh Report[1] quotes perceptions by individuals belonging to minorities of their career advancement in the NHS in these words:

> Black employees should feel lucky if they reach the status of ward or service managers as not many make it beyond that. While White managers feel that their rights to manage are well earned, Black managers are made to feel privileged when reaching that position. For many, the only way to grow into the job is through undying loyalty to those who pull the strings. Of course, that means distancing themselves from any blackness and to be seen to be tough on people of the same racial background so as to show that racial affinity is not going to get in their way. Frankly, it scares the hell out of me to see how divided we are among ourselves.

Even though individuals who appear outwardly different can find commonalities in other aspects of their lives. However, attitudes of prejudice, linked to superficial characteristics, can stop individuals from establishing meaningful relationships with someone who appears different at first sight. Such experiences of racism can be found among all ethnic categories, thereby confirming its relation to external appearance rather than immigration status. Experiences of racism further complicate the integration of migrants because it contributes to their exclusion.

There is some evidence that those nurses who migrated to Britain in the 1950s and 1960s have found it difficult to move into more senior positions; many remain in lower paid grades and job roles and the literature presents evidence of discriminatory practice hindering their progression.[2]

Even though most discriminatory attitudes may stem from the attitudes of a White majority towards a minority of ethnically diverse individuals, this is not always the case and there are also irregular aspects of racist attitudes. While prejudices that focus on race or ethnicity may primarily come from White colleagues, they can also be present among other Black and minority ethnic colleagues, reflecting the fact that racism has more faces than just skin colour, as noted by Parekh.

The following statement illustrates what is commonly seen as a 'typical' observation of racial discrimination:

> When we go in placement and they put you on duty with a White trainee nurse, the staff give that one [the White nurse] more attention than you, because they think you are Black and the ward sister is White.

In some cases a deeper change in underlying attitude among some 'White' senior staff is required for nurses from minority ethnic backgrounds to experience true equality and this cannot be accomplished through written policies.

Prejudices or 'prejudgements' are mostly not drawn on the basis of observed behaviour, but on the conclusions that individuals draw from what they see. For example, a British-trained nurse might observe an African nurse working at a different pace to him or herself, drawing the conclusion that they are 'lazy'. While some nurses from African countries may be happy to admit that they work differently, they would resent such a foregone conclusion. In fact they might express that they work in a more 'relaxed mode', which is not only more enjoyable but also creates less work-related stress.

It is difficult to assess to what extent claims that attitudes of discrimination towards non-British nurses directly and exclusively hinder their career progression. There are often a number of complex reasons why individuals do not progress, are unable to progress, or do not wish to progress in their careers. However, the fact that there is an unrepresentative high number of White, male managers in the NHS compared to a largely female and often non-White general workforce raises some questions about the fairness of the promotion processes in place.

Some managers express concern about some minority ethnic nurses using the 'racism argument' for their own lack of ambition, while some nurses who came to work in Britain 20 years ago have not progressed into senior nursing posts and they themselves blame racist attitudes towards them. To unravel all the complexities of racism goes beyond the scope of this book, but it certainly forms an important aspect along the journey towards integration.

The following migrant nurse had applied for a post in an Intensive Care Unit (ITU), a speciality with many unfilled vacancies, resulting in this particular unit having to keep a number of beds unused. After being refused for the post, the nurse felt puzzled and distressed and had this to say:

> I didn't get the post and I was very upset and I didn't find any valid reason why I was refused. For several nights I didn't sleep. There is nothing in my career profile that could be refused. About my head nurse, I am very sure that she has given a very good reference and I have worked here five years and in the past year I have not taken any sick leave. I can't think that I have been refused for professional reasons. Which means that if the government

here is trying to treat all the people the same way, there are still people here that don't treat all the people the same way.

While some migrant nurses experience such seemingly explicit discrimination, others observe that their colleagues are reluctant to change and develop their skills. Their lack of openness to embrace difference thus hinders the introduction of new and more inclusive procedures at the workplace.

At the same time, as Figures 6.1 and 6.2 above have indicated, many migrant nurses feel treated fairly and equally. A 45-year-old female nurse from Ghana who is a single parent with three children only had praise about how she was treated:

> My mentor is White, they are all English. I don't find any difference at all. I haven't experienced anything bad. There is no discrimination in my workplace.

Prejudices and the creation of perceived 'in-groups' and 'out-groups' create layers of social exclusion. Many individuals do not distinguish between different countries of origin of migrant workers and would not even be able to distinguish between people from African and Caribbean countries or different Eastern European origins. Yet they make sweeping statements about 'them' and 'all' being lazy or slow. Often such strong statements are the results of personal or collective feelings of anger and resentment, leading to the strong 'us and them' thinking typical of prejudice. Based on such underlying attitudes the 'other' will always remain an unknown entity, a non-person, and moreover the 'self' will not be scrutinised within the mirror of values that differ. Any such attitudes stifle organisational development even if policy statements embrace diversity, equal opportunities and fairness.

Even though racism deals specifically with prejudices related to skin colour and ethnicity, similar attitudes also translate to gender in relation to employment.

Meeting others: gender norms

Even on an international scale, nursing is a female-dominated career choice,[3] and with gender norms being culturally constructed, they vary from culture to culture. For example, the notion of 'otherness' commonly seems to include the expectation that women and particularly Muslim women act submissively. Consequently it may come as a surprise to some White, British-trained nurses that some women from a Muslim background can be outspoken, though others do indeed behave in a very reserved way.[4]

Stereotypical notions of masculinity seem to pressure men into some of the best-paying and most prestigious nursing specialities or management roles, therefore allowing male nurses to progress more easily. This seems to be confirmed when looking at male nurses' career progression. MacDougall[5] explains this by stating that while men often enter nursing for the same reasons as women, namely a desire to care for others, perceived job security and the power that accrues to a professional position, the pressure (from themselves or others) to conform to stereotypes of the 'dominant male' causes many to move away from caring roles into managerial positions.

Gender norms differ from country to country with further variations related to personal and family values. While some migrants to Britain state that 'it would be shameful for a woman to migrate by herself', others do not share such extreme views. Yet others feel misunderstood or even appalled, but unable to address gender-related behaviours in their British workplaces, as this female nurse from Somalia has encountered:

> This male nurse, when he is talking to you, he likes to put his arm around you.

While such behaviour may not reflect professional norms in British hospitals, the migrant nurse may nevertheless feel unable to address a male supervisor's sleazy behaviour.

When comparing responses given by male and female migrant nurses in the empirical questionnaire, there is no evidence of any correlation between gender and any current or previous clinical speciality, career progression or shift pattern. Yet the sample shows other gender-related differences.

- The majority of men (80% of all male respondents) were of Asian/Filipino origin, which nearly always meant that their employers had recruited them directly.
- The percentage of men who were financially supporting relatives outside the UK was slightly lower at 84% compared to 92% for women.
- Only five men (20% of all male respondents) had dependents living with them, compared to 44 of the women (38.3% of all female respondents).
- The female respondents had worked longer in their profession and nearly twice as long in their current post, the organisation and the NHS than the male respondents.
- When using t-tests to compare male and female nurses' responses, results showed that female respondents reported a higher perception of their organisation's implementation of equal opportunities policies and higher levels of support from both their supervisors and colleagues than the male respondents.

The fact that gender norms differ and the way this can be reflected in patient care becomes clear in the following statement, made by a migrant nurse who had spent some years working in Kuwait:

Actually, in Kuwait there would be no male and female patients on the same ward and you have male nurses for male patients. Here even though they are in different sides of the ward, it is more mixed and patients visit each other and sit on each other's beds. In Kuwait, if there is a male nurse we as female nurses should not be asked to look after the male patients, but here they don't care. I just try to be patient and get used to it.

Varying gender norms illustrate some of the adjustments migrants have to undergo when integrating into a very different employment context.

Migrants' perceptions of the implementation of equal opportunities policies, fairness and their own ability to be involved in their organisation are all indicators of their successful integration. Once migrants believe that they are treated equally and fairly, they can concentrate on their career and develop professionally without added worry about being treated less advantageously than their British-trained counterparts.

References

1   Parekh B (2000) *The Future of Multi-ethnic Britain: the Parekh report*. The Runnymede Trust, London.

2   Beishon S, Virdee S and Hagell A (1995) *Nursing in a Multi-ethnic NHS*. Policy Studies Institute, London.

3   Anker R (2001) *Gender and Jobs: sex segregation of occupations in the world*. International Labour Office, Geneva.

4   Summerfield H (1996) Patterns of adaptation: Somali and Bangladeshi women in Britain. In: G Buijs (ed) *Migrant Women, crossing boundaries and changing identities*. Berg, Oxford.

5   MacDougall G (1997) Caring – a masculine perspective. *Journal of Advanced Nursing*. **25**: 809–13.

CHAPTER 7

Integrating: meeting 'others' in their organisation

As was demonstrated in the previous chapters, relationships at work can increase individuals' identification with the work group and also with the wider organisation. Therefore increasing work-related identification can be symbolic of migrants' process of integrating into employment. Following on from some of the characteristics that mark out encounters with the 'other', this chapter highlights some of the milestones along the journey of integrating into the wider context of the employing organisation by tracing the journey in a chronological order, demonstrating some of the barriers and encounters along the way.

Entering and progressing in the organisation

Looking at the early stages of workplace integration, the difficulties for migrant nurses who have come to Britain independently of recruitment agencies need to be stressed. Unlike those nurses who are directly recruited, those who have come to Britain of their own accord face a range of barriers in adapting past training and experience to UK requirements.[1] In particular, many of the refugee nurses have not been able to work for several years following their arrival in Britain due to their immigration status or their personal circumstances, making them feel additionally vulnerable. Guidelines on how to adapt one's qualifications are available from the Nursing and Midwifery Council which holds the central register of all nurses registered in the UK.

One major hurdle is gaining access to a supervised practice placement, required by the Nursing and Midwifery Council in order to work as a registered nurse in Britain. Despite a national nursing shortage, there is strangely also a shortage of supervision placements for migrant nurses who did not arrive in cohorts. Moreover, some groups of internationally qualified nurses have paid thousands of pounds to access UK-based employment and have been recruited under false pretences to work in private care homes, doing no or very little clinical nursing. As a result many migrant nurses with years of experience end up working in the independent sector or as Health Care Assistants in care homes, neither being able to convert their qualifications nor being able to leave, as they often have to repay large debts incurred in order to finance their journey to Britain.

In addition to the practical and clinical hurdles to accessing supervision placements, there are often also added complications related to the migrants' immigration status as indicated above. Therefore some migrants and particularly those who are asylum seekers or refugees need to know who to turn to in confidence, should concerns about their Home Office status affect their employment. Knowing that such sensitive personal issues are treated with confidentiality inspires trust and also provides the migrant with the support needed should any problems regards their status arise.

On the one hand, the chronic shortage of supervision placements leaves many migrant nurses unable to find a hospital that will support their adaptation and enable them to become fully registered. On the other hand, other migrant nurses may have many years of practical experience, but due to differences in the training are unable to adapt their qualifications to UK-based standards. The following nurse from Moldova was such a case and she said:

> They ask, 'Why don't you start your adaptation?' I don't know, because I don't know anybody. I don't have anybody, you know. I talked to my manager in the care home, who didn't know that I only did two years of training and I explained that to her and showed her my papers. She said, 'Can I see your papers, maybe you didn't fill it out correctly?' I send back home for the transcript. I complained to the NMC to say it is not incomplete training and she helped me to write a letter. She wants me to do adaptation and to stay there, to work as a nurse. But it is very difficult to get a place for adaptation, but I would be happy to do that.

Due to the limited number of supervision placements available, migrant nurses tend to accept any that are offered to them, regardless of their aspirations to work in a particular clinical speciality or even geographical region in the UK. The following comment highlights what is a typical experience:

> We visited the Trust, we were not given a choice which speciality we could be because 'Care of the Elderly' were the only people who had accepted to take us on. We didn't have any choice. Yes, we had no choice, we had been waiting for a long time.

It is not uncommon for migrant nurses looking for a supervision placement to have written to hundreds of hospitals all over Britain, including Ireland and Scotland, and still not to have been offered a place. Managers give funding restrictions as one reason for not organising supervision placements, as funding for international recruitment is allocated from different sources compared to funding for independently run supervision courses for nurses already in the country. Other reasons may be a lack of available mentors or already overburdened management.

The completion of the supervision programme is a major stepping-stone in the migrants' integration process, giving them an incredible boost in self-confidence. This indicates a journey not only of development in professional capacity, but one that is experienced as positively shaping personal well-being on a wider scale, as comments from many other migrant nurses confirm:

> They try to trust me and let me control a patient by myself. Everything is fine and I am now quite happy.

> By the time I did three months, I got used to everything and people start to like me.

> I am much happier now, because I am confident.

> I feel confident that I am able to do the job as a trained staff nurse.

Feelings of happiness and improved well-being as result of increased trust by their colleagues commonly accompany the journey towards integration and act as intrinsic motivators to work. Increased feelings of confidence and personal happiness were symbolic of a turning point during the journey of integration. By this stage difficulties at work have been overcome and most migrant nurses start to perceive a sense of belonging.

One example given by a manager involved in the preparation of migrant nurses, and particularly refugees for NHS supervision programmes, demonstrates the effect of integration on the individual and also their wider personal space:

> Once she got into a job, the whole family would back her. They would all say, 'Now my mum has got a job, now when we go to school or college we can say, "My mum is a nurse" not "My mum is an unemployed nurse or on an English course" but "My mum is a nurse" and "She works at so-and-so." ' So it is the status of the whole family that gets raised, not just the individual.

This marked improvement in migrant nurses' general well-being once professional registration as a nurse is achieved even becomes physically observable. The same manager has observed a personal transition alongside migrant nurses' professional integration, marked by a change in body language and behaviour. She noted the following:

> Nine months later she got her PIN number and one of her tutors met her, she had to look at her twice because she looked so good. She had her hair done, she was walking straight. That nurse herself said: 'I am doing my job.' That's

it, that's all it was. She was the real person again, rather than the one that first came here, this rather sort of quiet, dowdy, shy and dull-looking person.

Becoming a registered nurse in Britain affirms migrants' personal and professional identity, often accompanied by feelings of achievement, confidence and pride. This also indicates that the individual nurses have managed to overcome the hurdles of gaining access to employment and those barriers associated with day-to-day work as a nurse in Britain. Yet it presents just the beginning of a nursing career in Britain.

Despite recent research stating that a high proportion of migrant nurses move on to other countries after having worked in Britain for a while,[2] there are also indications that those who have come here for non-work related reasons, such as refugees and people with families, are more likely to stay committed to working in the UK and working at the hospital that supported their integration.

When asked in the empirical survey how committed migrant nurses felt about staying at their current hospital, the typical response was: 'Yes, I feel committed, but I want to develop my career', indicating that commitment to the career is overriding commitment to the organisation. Therefore migrants, in the same way as other employees, are prepared to change employers where development into their chosen specialty is not possible in their current organisation. With most NHS employers offering study days, lectures or courses and nurses having to engage in personal development plans, there are some indications that career development is part of the wider organisational agenda. In practice, however, this may not be quite as apparent.

The survey data allow comparison between migrant nurses' levels of commitment to the immediate workgroup, their career and the employing organisation. When comparing the mean of organisational, occupational and workgroup commitment (measured on a 7-point Likert scale with 1 being low and 7 high commitment), mean occupational commitment was 5.34, higher than mean organisational commitment (5.30) and workgroup commitment (5.10):

Table 7.1   Mean and standard deviation work-related commitment

	Type of commitment	*Mean*	*Standard deviation*
1	Organisational commitment	5.30	(1.20)
2	Occupational/career commitment	5.43	(1.10)
3	Workgroup commitment	5.10	(1.16)

These findings confirm migrant nurses' strong commitment to their professional career. Even though some employees feel that their personal identity benefits from belonging to an 'in-group'[3] and they might therefore be very dedicated to their workgroup, yet overall, workgroup commitment was reported as being comparatively lower.

Professional identity with the chosen career can be an integral part of personal identity, as this manager has observed in some of the migrant nurses employed by her hospital:

> Some of the migrant nurses have said to me they couldn't envisage to do anything else. An alternative employment other than healthcare was not even something they could contemplate. Therefore one of the things we are looking at is an accelerated promotion process because we want to build on the experience that some of these migrant nurses have.

With nursing being so integral to individuals, career aims and objectives should be discussed in a two-way dialogue and consultation process between the individual nurse and a mentor or supervisor. The individual determines career-related interests in an autonomous way and, following discussions, has these supported by the organisation. Such an approach to career development serves a range of purposes.

- It encourages the individual by valuing their personal preferences and skills.
- It should encourage retention and decrease turnover.
- It keeps the workforce up to date on the latest clinical developments, thus providing the most advanced nursing care possible.

Thus career commitment is directly linked to organisational commitment and where professional career development is not supported and implemented by the managers of the organisation in practice this can hinder individual growth and also identification with that workplace:

> The Trust is supportive, but the ward managers are the hindrance to our growth, as they don't give us the opportunities announced to us.

As with most organisational policies, career development plans need to be implemented and supported from the top down to the day-to-day managers and colleagues to be truly effective.

The organisation and non-work-related responsibilities

Associations between non-work-related commitments, such as caring responsibilities for family members and work-related commitments, can affect integration and also well-being at work. Caring responsibilities can take the form of sending money to support family members who live outside Britain or having to bring up and care for children while working full-time and trying to integrate into employment in Britain (*see* Table 3.3 for how common this was among the survey respondents in the empirical study).

Many nurses, including British-qualified ones, have to juggle multiple commitments and take care of home- and work-related responsibilities. However, to do this within an unfamiliar country and work setting can cause additional pressures and the way in which some migrants are coping confirms their dedication to both work and family. The following refugee nurse from Rwanda, for example, while looking after four children at home, was amongst the first to be promoted within a year of having received her registration:

> Nursing has been part of my life and that's my job since a long time ago. I don't think I can change and I have a family and I need to find my way to survive and to support my children. It's new, we are trying to adapt to everything. This is new for us. When I am at work they are at school. The children, sometimes the eldest will pick up the youngest; the young one is $3\frac{1}{2}$ years old, he is still very small.

Despite an obvious tension associated with looking after school-aged children and working full time, very few migrant nurses, and nurses in general, take up an opportunity to work part time. With high costs of living, even though working part-time may give nurses more flexibility, many are not able to meet their financial commitments on a part-time salary. Thus, like their British counterparts, some migrants find themselves trapped between their reproductive and productive roles in society.

The empirical survey asked respondents if:

1   they had dependants living with them and
2   they were financially supporting relatives outside Britain (*see* Table 3.3).

These demographic characteristics formed the basis for the comparison of work-related types of commitments, such as commitment to the workgroup, the professional career or the organisation, leading to some interesting results: findings showed first that levels of organisational commitment were higher among those nurses who had dependants living with them and second, that those who lived with dependants reported lower levels of work-related stress. This may come as a surprise, as one public assumption seems to be that 'working parents' are more stressed than those who do not have any children.

One explanation of these findings is that nurses with an economic responsibility for their families rely more on a regular income and thus may express this in strong organisational commitment, which could be 'continuance commitment'.[4] In other words nurses feel committed to the organisation because they rely on the security this provides.

This is confirmed when the migrant nurses further explain how they feel about the organisation. Comments made are that they appreciate the 'security employment offered' and the 'good financial support' they receive through working.

Other empirical findings show that 25% of the survey sample sent money outside the UK to support relatives, as well as having dependants living with them in Britain. Those who did, reported higher levels of commitment to their career, pointing to a personal identification with the nursing profession and a personal drive to better one's prospects. The same group of respondents also reported a more positive perception of their organisation's innovation and effectiveness, higher levels of work-related happiness and a stronger intention to stay with the organisation.

This confirms a positive relationship between personal responsibilities and commitment to the organisation as well as general well-being at work. Personal identities related to family and relatives seem to enhance positively how individuals feel about their employing organisation: there seems to be a correlation between financial responsibilities for family members and positive feelings about work. Consequently, even if some nurses stay with an organisation as a result of socio-economic pressure, they will not necessarily be unhappy in their workplace or perceive their organisation as a negative place to be.

References

1   Eversley J and Watts H (2001) *Refugee and Overseas Qualified Nurses Living in the UK*. Praxis and Queen Mary and Westfield, University of London, London.

2   Buchan J, Jobanputra R and Gough P (2005) Should I stay or should I go? A survey from the Kings Fund and RCN. *Nursing Standard*. **19**(36): 14–16.

3   Hogg MA and Terry DJ (2000) Social identity and self-categorization processes in organizational contexts. *Academy of Management Review*. **25**(1): 121–40.

4   Meyer JP and Allen NJ (1997) *Commitment in the Workplace: theory, research and application*. SAGE, London.

CHAPTER 8

Contributing: the contribution of migrant nurses

The contribution migrant nurses are making to organisations in Britain rests on the concepts of diversity management and capacity building. To start with, the theoretical concept and practical application of diversity within the workforce is currently receiving considerable attention in the literature. With greater acceptance of labour mobility, mergers and market expansions, corporations are becoming more and more multinational, resulting in an increasingly mixed workforce.[1] Increased demographic diversity is also the result of increased international migration and the implementation of equal opportunities policies in the UK.[2] However, the implications of diversity for management are not restricted to a drive towards equal opportunity quotas and the representation of the local community within the workforce in numerical terms.[3] The United Nations defined diversity in the following way:[4]

> Diversity takes many forms. It is usually thought of in terms of obvious attributes – age, race, gender, physical ability, sexual orientation, religion and language. Diversity in terms of background professional experience, skills and specialisation, values and culture, as well as social class, is a prevailing pattern.

This definition, like others, distinguishes between deep-level (attitudinal) and surface-level (demographic) diversity.[5-7] The deeper layer to diversity encompasses attitudes, values, religion, beliefs, lifestyles and identities, invisible and often only known to the beholder. By contrast, surface-level diversity concentrating on demographic differences can in organisations also include employment related aspects, for instance occupation, organisational status and ability.[8]

Employees not only originate from a variety of demographic backgrounds, but also hold divergent underlying belief systems. Such obvious and hidden facets of personal identity affect how individuals relate to each other at work, how they communicate, what kind of attitudes and behaviours they display and how these influence group cohesion and integration. It is dangerous, there-fore, to stereotype individuals based on the demographic aspects of diversity. For example, the category 'Black' can include people of numerous regional origins, such as Caribbean, African, Asian or European British.[9] At the same time individuals can group themselves and gravitate towards existing communities which display very different types of behaviour. For example, Summerfield[10] found that following migration to London Somali women were more in control of their lives and integrated more easily than women from Bangladesh. Yet for any outsider to assume certain behaviour patterns on the basis that someone is of Bangladeshi or Somali origin would be wrong.

The increase in diversity has led to a body of research which looks at its effects on organisational behaviour, such as productivity, conflict and group socialisation and management implications.[11] Studies have established that a diverse workgroup with a wider range of ideas and experiences can be more productive in tasks which require creativity and judgement.[12-13] To achieve this, strong workgroup commitment is required, which can be reached through bringing people together, clear communication and clarity in objectives and decision making.[14] Yet problems in communication and social integration can affect commitment to the team and lead to a lack of identification with the group's goals. As a result sub-groups can develop, conflicts arise and communication can break down.[12]

Such antagonism can be prevented through careful management of the group, especially during the early, formative stages. Watson et al.[13] imply that group socialisation, provided it is managed constructively, could have positive long-term consequences for organisations, overriding the problems associated with differences. Watson et al. go on to stress that in order to achieve these positive group outcomes, managers need to provide the group with regular assessments and feedback on performance and group processes. As a result, group members can be encouraged to discuss how things are going and how problems could be addressed.

If such constructive management does not take place, Blau[15] and O'Reilly et al.[16] state that demographic diversity decreases social contacts, as individuals naturally relate to others whom they perceive as similar, thus reducing social integration, leading to low workgroup commitment. Therefore demographic heterogeneity can hamper the process of group formation and attitudes of stereotyping and prejudice can lead to in- and out-groups.[17] This can be reflected in the levels of commitment to and identification with the wider organisation.[18]

Intolerance and discrimination can directly affect social identification within groups as well as commitment to groups, and indirectly they affect work outcomes such as turnover, performance and communication. This emphasises the importance of the concepts of work-related motivation and emotions at work and these can shed light on some of the underlying dynamics of the employment context, such as the aspects of work which individuals enjoy and receive satisfaction from. The correlation between work effectiveness and diversity among workers is reliant on mediating factors, such as supportive management, clear work goals and open communication, and this can also be exacerbated by an organisation's culture.

Effective organisational management approaches consider the organisation's aim, often expressed in mission statements of which the following – of a London-based NHS hospital – is a typical example:

> Keeping the people of [place] in the best of health – caring for our community, our staff and our hospital. To do this we will: provide the best possible quality services, have close links with the community, continue the pursuit of clinical excellence, expand our academic teaching and research base.

Together with the national NHS strategy they point to the organisation aiming to achieve congruence between the internal organisational structures and procedures and the organisational environment in order to achieve specific results. Ultimately each organisation needs to define worthwhile internal and external organisational outcomes for itself, with inputs from its employees and users, stressing the importance for a context-specific definition of organisational effectiveness.

By applying the concept of capacity building to migrant nurses' contribution to a British organisation, the stereotypical 'North to South' exchange of knowledge and expertise is being challenged. Even though the concept of capacity building has its roots in international development, organisations worldwide utilise the individual competencies and capabilities of their members to increase their effectiveness.

Individual competence or *capability* is the 'ability or skill to do something, to understand and learn or to do or produce',[19] the distinctive contribution made by individuals to the organisation or the rest of the team. Therefore even though managers attempt to direct the organisational behaviour of staff, it is down to the individual to make a difference and to contribute to organisational capacity.[20]

The concept of capacity embraces a range of organisational dimensions[21] and in order to develop capacity the organisation has to reach congruence between internal organisational behaviour, such as management structures aimed to motivate employees, and its external aims and objectives.[22-5] Organisational change in response to changes in the environment and the needs of service recipients is required in order to improve capacity. Such changes could include changes in recruitment strategy to address staff shortages or to achieve a workforce that is ethnically representative of the local population, with consequences for the way diversity is managed in practice. Achieving this can be a difficult process in large, bureaucratic organisations as they tend to find it more difficult than smaller organisations with fewer layers in the hierarchy to correct behaviour and learn from errors. Yet not being able to adjust to changing client demands and a changing environment stifles an organisation.[26-9]

A key policy debate in the NHS is focused currently on capacity, with the challenges of balancing limited financial resources with performance targets.[30] Capacity building as a concept is about more than resources, especially in the healthcare sector, where relationships between staff and clients are the key to success.[31] Therefore approaches to capacity building need to take employee motivation and concepts of identity into account. This is especially crucial when the workforce is composed of individuals from diverse backgrounds, including refugees as one sub-group of internationally qualified nurses.[32-4]

For individual migrant nurses to contribute their individual capabilities to overall organisational capacity, the NHS as a whole and the employing healthcare trusts need to manage diverse work teams constructively. Successful management of diversity is reflected in relationships at work, positive work-related emotions and work-related identities; issues discussed in the previous chapters. These in turn can lead to committed employees who are more inclined to engage in organisational citizenship behaviour which is discretionary and a matter of choice[35] and contribute their skills and knowledge to the organisation.[36-7]

The NHS organisational capacity objectives are set out in the government's reform agenda, with some of the key points being an expansion in staff numbers and a redesign of jobs by creating smaller, integrated teams. In part the government plans to meet these objectives through improving staff morale and building people management skills.[38] Achieving capacity within organisations is to a degree derived from 'effective management of people, their commitment to and involvement with the organisation'.[14] Within multicultural organisations the successful management of diversity seems to be the basis for capacity.

The survey data in the empirical study showed that most respondents perceived their organisation as slightly more effective than innovative and perceived their promotion opportunities as quite high. Thus even though organisations may be viewed as performing effectively, their openness to change, reflected in innovation was not seen as quite as high:

Table 8.1 Nurses' perceptions of the organisation

Variable	Mean	Standard deviation
Organisational effectiveness	4.69	(1.15)
Organisational innovation	4.49	(1.14)
Promotion opportunity	5.31	(1.33)

Further analysis showed that respondents' perceptions of organisational effectiveness were the result of a combination of personal identities, namely feelings of happiness at work, commitment to the organisation and workgroup, and managerial factors (the management of equal opportunities and supervisor support) – confirming that human resource components are a key factor in achieving organisational capacity.

Box 8.1 Personal and managerial factors related to capacity

Personal factors:

- Feeling of happiness at work
- Commitment to the workgroup
- Commitment to the organisation

Managerial factors:

- Management of equal opportunities
- Support received from supervisors

This also reflects in the personal accounts given by migrant nurses and their managers about the contribution newcomers are making to existing work-groups and the wider organisational objectives. This section commences with positive expressions of migrant nurse's contributions before going on to some of the obstacles to them contributing.

Positive expressions of migrant nurses contributing

When asked how they would describe their personal contribution to the wider workgroup, the following remarks are typical examples of how migrant nurses view the value they are adding:

I share my previous experience.

I am a good team player, motivated, give encouragement and support to my colleagues.

I cover for colleagues on holiday or sick leave or [when we are] short of staff, I help other teams when necessary.

I am supportive, caring, enthusiastic.

I am honest and have a good sense of humour.

I am dedicating my whole life to the patients, to the management, to the ward to run smoothly.

The contribution of past professional experience, to a current job may seem logical. In some cases though past experience can differ greatly from what is expected in a current job, leading to a difficult transition for the individual. To be co-operative and supportive to colleagues in the work team may not explicitly be stated in an employment contract, but is an essential aspect of capacity as it 'oils the wheels' of the organisation, also called pro-social organisational behaviour or organisational citizenship behaviour. Such contributions to the functioning of the work team are likely to strengthen workgroup commitment.

As pointed out above, there are key stages in the integration process which are accompanied by a range of emotions, with migrants reporting that they feel more *confident* and *trusted* once they are granted their registration with the Nursing and Midwifery Council.

The following comment made by a 28-year-old nurse from Moldova illustrates the progression from the ignored newcomer to the trusted professional whose opinion is valued by other team members:

In the beginning it was really hard, they don't trust you. I tell them I am a nurse, but they ignored me. I thought it was because of my English. Little by little I started to say my opinion about diagnosis and tried to make conversation. After six months they started to ask me, 'What is your opinion?'

Therefore contributing to capacity is a process marked out by the newcomer feeling more positive about language, the employment context, relationships and their own confidence to contribute as they integrate with integration being a two-way process whereby British-trained nurses also get to know the 'stranger' and show an interest in her or his opinion and experience. The examples presented are based on migrants experiencing this process of inclusion.

Contributing individual capabilities to the workgroup and wider organisation can take many forms. While some duties are expressed in professional codes of conduct, many are not and rest on individuals taking initiative. The list of how individuals enhance their workplaces is endless and the following are just a few examples:

- volunteering to cover for colleagues who are ill
- showing an ambition in learning new procedures
- translating for medical staff or patients
- applying past teaching experience by mentoring junior healthcare staff
- contributing cultural knowledge related to patient care in a cross-cultural setting
- viewing accountability as an incentive to enhance personal knowledge.

Cultural understanding

The following quote was made by a migrant nurse who had worked in a Muslim country leading her to view patients' privacy as important, something that is also part of the British approach to nursing. Her manner of working ensures strict personal privacy, something that is valued by her manager, who may know that not all the nurses adhere to similar standards:

> The manager I worked with was very happy when I washed a patient, because I kept the privacy all the time, because I was used to it already. Even giving the commode, some of the nurses don't close the curtains, just give the commode and it is in full view of the other patients. Then there was a patient and she was changing her bra. I came and closed the curtains to give her privacy, but her response was, 'Oh, nurse, I don't mind.'

Many migrant nurses, particularly from African countries, are used to working very independently, in rural areas, often being one of only a few healthcare professionals accessible to the population. They therefore have to carry out tasks that only a medical doctor would do in a Western country. Yet they are not allowed to utilise some of these skills in the British NHS, which has strict professional boundaries. Instead of getting frustrated, successful integration into the work team is signified by an acceptance of the differences in the way healthcare systems operate. This nurse from the Congo had adopted such attitude:

> In Congo they carry out the task allocated to the doctor, but here the nurse is accountable for his action. The nurse must be very careful in practice, but it helped me to develop myself and it is a motivation for me to learn more and to assure good practice.

Working as part of a diverse team, migrant nurses can sometimes offer a new perspective on routine practices. With Filipino nurses in particular being recruited in high numbers on some hospital wards, they can have a real influence on the work-culture there. An NHS human resources manager whose hospital employs high numbers of migrant nurses directly recruited from the Philippines, conducted an analysis of patients' complaints about nursing care. He concluded that none related to Filipino nurses:

> 80–90% of complaints by patients are around attitudes of staff, generally nursing staff. Some of this may be related to cultural differences in some way. But there is no problem with the Filipino nurses, and no complaint has ever been made about them.

Other managers point to the 'American approach' to nursing brought by many of the Filipino nurses who had already migrated from the Philippines to Saudi Arabia before coming to the UK. This process of multiple exposure to different cultures in itself makes them more adaptable to different organisational settings.

Yet others confirmed that the recruitment of Filipino nurses has a measurable impact on the way their hospital is managed. For example, in the case of St. Mary's NHS Healthcare Trust in London, the change in recruitment policy away from employing expensive agency nurses towards recruiting large numbers of full-time nurses from the Philippines, has, according to Osborne[39] led to improvements in patient care as well as staff morale. Overall the hospital progressed from a one-star rating to a three-star rating and Osborne concluded that large-scale international recruitment could have a positive effect on organisational capacity, at least in the short term. This not only had a positive impact on vacancy figures and turnover, but also released financial resources for other needs.

Another form of contributing culturally is by the usage of languages spoken by migrants. Most of them speak more than one language with English commonly being their second or third language. When qualified translators are not at hand, colleagues and doctors frequently draw on the migrant nurses' multiple language skills. For a minority of patients the ability of a nurse to be able to communicate with them in their mother tongue plays a distinctive role in helping them to trust the healthcare they receive, thus aiding recovery.

Organisational citizenship behaviour

Getting to know colleagues, and starting to feel more confident within the British nursing system can be motivating to practice organisational citizenship behaviour, and thereby contribute to smooth running of the organisation. Employees decide to contribute above the written obligations, 'to go beyond the call of duty' which can take a range of forms from being concerned about colleagues' well-being to spending extra time with concerned patients or organising informal training sessions for junior staff.

Strong intrinsic motivation can led to nurses investing their private time to develop their professional knowledge, ultimately using this to advance their careers as well as contributing to organisational objectives. The following example was given by a migrant nurse from Ghana who wanted to develop her skills related to administrative tasks, documenting patient care which form part of her nursing job:

> On my day off, if I was at home, I sometimes called them, asking 'Should I come today?' Just, you know, to be in the office, to learn one or two things in the office.

Organisational citizenship behaviour can also draw on migrants' previous experience. For example by using previous clinical, managerial or teaching experience to facilitate others' professional development. Even though the following nurse did not immediately receive formal acknowledgement in the form of promotion and a pay increase, she later went on to train as a mentor, and teaching others comes naturally to her as a result of her past experience:

> On our ward we have a number of Health Care Assistants, who are on a pre-registration course. So they need a mentor and I help them, because I used to teach in a School of Nursing in Rwanda.

To take such initiatives reflects commitment to the organisation and ones colleagues, but it also confirms a strong professional career commitment, adapting skills gained in the past in order to benefit the current organisation. It also becomes clear that professional development is not something that should be left to managers to organise and even newcomers are called to take initiative in shaping their professional future, however foreign the professional culture may still seem.

Professional experience

The fact that many migrant nurses bring many years of professional experience with them was confirmed by some of the hospital managers' comments in the empirical study. Managers pointed out that internationally qualified nurses are very experienced nurses and once they have done their supervised practice programme, they are able to function quickly as fully registered nurses. Unlike newly qualified nurses, migrant nurses are mature individuals who don't need to be shown how to do basic nursing tasks.

When asked about the capacity that migrant nurses were adding to the hospitals, managers highlighted several dimensions. First, past experience is seen as an asset. One manager gave an example of a nurse's past experience of treating patients with Tuberculosis (TB), a disease on the increase in Britain, particularly in London:

> We have some migrant nurses who have come from South Africa. They now work in the TB service and obviously their experience of TB in Africa and TB here adds to the breadth of support that can be given.

Second, managers noted the personal attributes and emotional strengths that migrant nurses and particularly some of the refugee nurses bring to the organisation. These attributes reflect in motivation and leadership skills on the ward:

> I don't know if it is because of their refugee status, but they are a very, very vocal group. They are very good practitioners and they are very keen,

very motivated. They provide very good leadership on the ward. You know we are very lucky to have them.

Third, the professional experience of many migrant nurses also reflects in their cultural understanding as pointed out above and the value they add to a diverse workforce is examined next.

Adding diversity

As noted above, access to employment for internationally qualified nurses who migrate independently of recruitment agencies is more difficult than for directly recruited nurses. Many migrants in this sub-group come to Britain for non-nursing related reasons and may not have undertaken clinical duties for a number of years. In addition, family commitments may have inhibited full-time work and others may not be aware of employment routes into nursing. Thus some of these nurses may need to refresh their clinical skills in addition to adapting to British nursing ethics. Some managers are aware of these additional burdens on migrant nurses and the following example of a change in hospital recruitment policies outlines the long-term organisational benefits of support- ing nurses who are already settled within Britain and intend to stay here:

> Our Trust has consciously made the decision to view the local population in terms of filling our vacancies and more so in terms of staff retention. From our research of why staff leave, we know that they can't stay any more in our local area because of housing, they often don't have their friends and London is an unknown area. So we made the decision generally to try to recruit locally. And actually one of the strategies of our recruitment and retention policy is to train our own people. So we are looking at people within the com- munity, developing their skills, developing their confidence to apply for Health Care Assistant positions, then train them to have the skills to go for a nursing profession.
>
> Previously, a year to 18 months ago, we have done an overseas recruit- ment campaign in the Philippines and followed government guidelines. We have supported 60 overseas nurses to adapt to the culture and the NHS. Because they are qualified nurses, they don't need any additional nursing input, but they need that adaptation process. That went very successfully, but in view of our local strategy about local employment and elements of the number of applications that have local addresses, we decided to tap into that. So we made a conscious decision not to recruit actively from abroad. Recently we had a big campaign and we advertised and we reviewed all our applications, we kept it to the London area and from that we actually had 159 applicants, that was then shortlisted down.

Direct recruitment from the Philippines may appear to be just as successful, as these nurses' up-to-date nursing experience enables them to adapt quickly. Yet it has to be stressed that in order to retain recruited staff, a recruitment strategy is needed, encouraging migrant nurses who already live in Britain to integrate into healthcare employment.

Another example of such a strategy is that of Guy's and St Thomas' NHS Hospital Trust in London, which launched a major local recruitment campaign in early 2003 to help the Trust's workforce to better reflect the diversity of the local community.[40] The argument of reflecting the local community in which the healthcare service operates is strongly advocated by employers and voluntary or community organisations. Often the ethnicity of the NHS workforce does not represent the ethnic mix of diverse communities and it is a well documented difficulty to attract for example Bangladeshis or Pakistanis into nursing. Employing more nurses from diverse backgrounds is therefore seen as adding real value to the organisation:

> I think also the value for me is supporting people who want to make their home in East London. I think the Trust has a commitment as the largest local employer. Our Chief Executive is committed to employ local people and it is quite popular at the moment. It is more about supporting people in the profession they choose and bringing them into the health service.

Thus migrant nurses are appreciated as employees because of their professionalism based on past working experience and personal maturity as well as the diversity they add to work teams.

Problems associated with migrant nurses contributing

Some of the obstacles migrant nurses face when trying to integrate into British healthcare employment are illustrated above. Some of these hindrances are overcome as the nurses adapted, but others can still pose a stumbling block for the nurses to contribute to the best of their abilities.

Problems related to cultural differences and diversity

A lecturer involved in teaching migrant nurses described some of the cross-cultural problems that refugee nurses in particular encounter during the early phases of their journey of adaptation to British nursing practice:

This nurse was struggling because he or she was a refugee and was in a war area. So the objective was that they save lives, irrespectively of where dignity comes in or respect comes in. In a war-torn area you don't think 'Oh, I should cover the patient with a blanket when I do a bed-bath. I need to ensure privacy' or whatever. For them to come to this country and practise differently takes time. He has no concept how to handle a bed-bath with dignity and respect and thereby it conflicts with UK nursing.

Aspects such as ensuring privacy are important as they define a contribution to quality of care. Yet many migrant nurses have in the past worked in systems that were lacking finances, equipment and reference books, leading to different standards in hygiene, privacy and the range of tasks carried out by qualified nurses. Such working environments with fewer regulations can also lead to the nurses being met with more respect than they get in Britain.

With a large aspect of the organisational effectiveness of hospitals being measured on the patient's satisfaction with the care they receive, developing skills of effective cross-cultural communication between nurse and patient are a direct contribution to capacity building.[41] As was noted above in relation to work-related relationships, particularly in the beginning some migrant nurses experience lack of trust or respect from patients. They find that similarly to some colleagues, patients also find it difficult to distinguish between professional competence and superficial attributes such as language skills and skin colour:

What can I say if the English nurses speak very good English? I think the patients can trust them more, unless they see our experience and then can trust us too.

Managing a diverse work team means overcoming those communication problems among staff as well as with patients as cross-cultural misunderstandings can escalate if no effort is made to really understand what the meaning behind certain words is. A manager gave this illustration of how cultural miscommunication can have far-reaching consequences on another's well-being, in this case the patient's:

A young man in his 20s came in for relatively minor surgery. The nurse on night shift was a Nigerian nurse and was doing the round and noticed that he wasn't sleeping and said to him 'What's the matter with you?' and he said, 'Well, actually' – and he had been psyching himself up to say this all day – 'I am really scared about tomorrow.' And what she said to him was, 'Don't be such a big baby, go to sleep now.' And he was devastated by it and at the time I think he felt very small indeed. After the surgery he thought about it and he was quite angry about it and it became a formal complaint.

The nurse had behaved in the way that was expected of her in Nigeria, but it had upset this British patient immensely. Subsequently her perceived lack of ability to offer support to the patient led to questions about her professional capabilities in Britain, yet it was an issue of miscommunication.

The cultural differences also become apparent as they interrelate with professional standards and diversity issues.

Problems related to professional nursing

Despite their many years of experience, some internationally qualified nurses feel that the nursing policies and procedures in Britain are so different that they have little to contribute. Moreover, migrant nurses can resent the fact that additional training is required of them in order to be able to conduct certain procedures, particularly where this relates to procedures such as intravenous catheterisation which many have carried out routinely in other countries:

> Oh my God, those policies, some I don't know, we are not given time to read the policies. They relate to any nursing task, it is also something of a barrier. Every time you do something like IV and catheterisation, you go and read up. Here they say I have to go for training, but I did that back home.

Thus institutional hurdles to full professional integration can remain even after migrant nurses have gained access to employment and registration. Although there may be professional justification, such as maintaining nursing standards for these policies and procedures, they can appear suffocating to some migrant nurses who may be more used to practical hands-on procedures than to written policies.

The British healthcare system also gives more power to patients than some of the migrants were used to and nurses in Britain are held to be more accountable than may be the case in some developing countries. This leads to a fear of litigation and disciplinary action among all groups of nurses but particularly newcomers to the system. Yet patient's rights can also inhibit their rate of recovery if they do not move from dependency to helping themselves.

From the patient's point of view legislation helps to ensure that they are being cared for and given the power to be proactive if they are not satisfied with any aspect of their care. For migrant nurses this type of working environment often differs greatly from what they were used to. Thus some nurses need more time and management support to get used to this 'patient-empowered' working environment. Such differences in nursing tasks are closely related to different nursing roles in Britain compared to other countries and can be perceived to undermine competencies.

For example, elements of personal care, such as washing and feeding patients, are in some countries either done by care assistants or by the patient's relatives. Yet British nursing ethics regard these tasks as part of patient care undertaken by nurses (even though practice may differ from this idealistic approach in many UK hospitals). Such tasks may resemble for some migrant nurses a direct extension of the reproductive, caring role of women,[42,43] which differs from the professional status they experienced in the past:

> In Bulgaria, in the hospital, the nurse don't wash the patients. I studied for three years to be a nurse. I not studied to wash the patients.

A lecturer involved in the running of adaptation programmes confirmed that the NHS nursing tasks sometimes conflict with those that many internationally qualified nurses are familiar with. He emphasised the basic nursing responsibilities criticised in the above comment, as important contributions to comprehensive nursing:

> If you are a staff nurse you can do the basic things. But it is not the basic things that are important, but the ability to analyse the situation. If you bath a patient you don't just do that, but you observe the patient for any bruises, cuts, bleeding, anything. And it is the contact with the patient, bathing, talking etc. that gives you the confidence. The patient may be depressed and if you just bath them, you miss all that. If you are adapting you need to learn that area.

This indicates an individual's need for support, communication and feeling accepted particularly during the early stages while newcomers try to understand their new workplace and try to figure out how they can best contribute. It also implies that managers should be prepared to review practice in light of what migrant nurses who have worked in different healthcare systems have to add and thus the establishment of open communication systems is fundamental. An unwillingness on behalf of managers to reflect and be open to changing policies and procedures can not only hamper migrants' integration, but moreover organisational development. A female refugee nurse from Africa said:

> We can't progress with all those problems on the ward. The ward manager is very reluctant to change, he doesn't discuss problems.

Some migrant nurses clearly make suggestions for improvement, but some feel that their suggestions are ignored, or that their colleagues are not truly open to be challenged.

Problems with the retention of migrant nurses

A desired organisational outcome of recruitment, professional development, promotion and management support for the migrant nurses is that they subsequently choose to stay with the organisation out of their own free will, not because there are no alternatives. With recruitment as well as the retention of trained nurses being a problem for many NHS trusts, especially in urban areas, 'nurses staying with the organisation' is considered an important organisational goal. Some nurses may continue working, but with less overall job satisfaction and with a lower level of 'affective' commitment: for example, nurses may stay because of a lack of alternative employment but not because they are really happy with the organisation.[44] In order to determine possible precursors of an individual's tendency to stay or to quit a current job, Mobley *et al.*[45] introduced the topic of employees' turnover and the intention to quit a particular job. This work was followed by further theoretical contributions on 'job satisfaction' and 'organisational commitment' which were found to be relevant antecedents to employee turnover.[46–50]

Table 8.2 demonstrates that levels of job satisfaction among the empirical survey respondents were reported as slightly higher than the intention to stay with the organisation, which could indicate that internationally qualified nurses would stay within their profession, even if they change the employing organisation:

Table 8.2 Intention to stay and job satisfaction

Variable	Mean	Standard deviation
Job satisfaction	4.99	(1.20)
Intention to leave/stay	4.78	(1.45)

Therefore high levels of experienced job satisfaction do not necessarily lead to individuals wanting to stay with the organisation that employs them. There may be other reasons for wanting to stay, such as migrants feeling settled in the area where their hospital is situated.

Several NHS managers are now realising that the direct overseas recruitment of migrant nurses to fill existing staffing vacancies is only a short-term solution, with many not wanting to settle in Britain, as this manager has experienced:

> From a retention point of view, it is probably positive. Those Swedish nurses will probably only stay a few years and the Australian, New Zealand nurses, but some of the other nurses who live in the local area will add value by staying.

The retention of migrant nurses, however, has been much debated in the recent press. Hall wrote in the *Telegraph* that four out of ten nurses from abroad are planning to leave London for other jobs. In particular two-thirds of nurses directly recruited from the Philippines are said to be planning to migrate on to America, which is also recruiting nurses for its staff shortages.[51,52] Thus the employment of migrant nurses who came independently of work and intend to stay in Britain offers comparatively more real value from a recruitment point of view.

References

1 Palma-Rivas N (2000) Current status of diversity initiative in selected multinational corporations. *Human Resource Development Quarterly*. **11**(1): 35–52.

2 Liff S (1999) Diversity and equal opportunities: room for constructive compromise? *Human Resource Management Journal*. **9**(1): 65–75.

3 Milliken FJ and Martins LL (1996) Searching for common treats: understanding the multiple effects of diversity in organisational groups. *Academy of Management Review*. **21**(2): 402–33.

4 United Nations (2000) Definition of diversity. In: P Clements and J Jones (ed) *The Diversity Training Handbook*. Kogan Page Limited, London.

5 Tajfel H and Turner JC (1979) Social groups and identities. In: WP Robinson (ed) *Developing the Legacy of Henry Tajfel*. Butterworth-Heinemann, Oxford.

6 Harrison DA, Price KH and Bell MP (1998) Beyond relational demography: time and the effects of surface- and deep- level diversity on work group cohesion. *Academy of Management Journal*. **41**(1): 96–107.

7 Lau DC and Murnighan JK (1998) Demographic diversity and faultlines: the compositional dynamics of organisational groups. *Academy of Management Review*. **23**(2): 325–40.

8 Larkey LK (1996) Towards a theory of communicative interactions in culturally diverse workgroups. *Academy of Management Review*. **21**(2): 463–91.

9 Kirton G and Greene A-M (2000) *The Dynamics of Managing Diversity: a critical approach*. Butterworth-Heinemann, London.

10 Summerfield H (1996) Patterns of adaptation: Somali and Bangladeshi women in Britain. In: G Buijs (ed) *Migrant Women: crossing boundaries and changing identities*. Berg, Oxford.

11 Cox TH, Lobel SA and McLeod PL (1991) Effects of ethnic group cultural differences on cooperative and competitive behaviour on a group task. *Academy of Management Journal*. **34**(4): 827–47.

12 Chatman JA, Polzer JT, Barsade SG *et al.* (1998) Being different yet feeling similar: the influence of demographic composition and organisational culture on work processes and outcomes. *Administrative Science Quarterly*. **43**: 749–80.

13 Watson WE, Kumar K and Michaelsen LK (1993) Cultural diversity's impact on interaction process and performance: comparing homogenous and diverse task groups. *Academy of Management Journal*. **36**(3): 590–602.

14 Mullins LJ (2002) Managerial behaviour and effectiveness. In: LJ Mullins (ed) *Management and Organisational Behaviour* (6e). Prentice Hall, London.

15 Blau P (1977) *Inequality and Heterogeneity*. Free Press, New York.

16 O'Reilly CA, Caldwell DF and Barnett WP (1989) Work group demographic, social integration, and turnover. *Administrative Science Quarterly*. **34**: 21–37.

17 Tsui AS, and O'Reilly CA (1989) Beyond simple demographic effects: the importance of relational demographic in superior-subordinate dyads. *Academy of Management Journal*. **32**(2): 402–23.

18 Mathieu JE and Zajac DM (1990) A review and meta-analysis of the antecedents, correlates and consequences of organisational commitment. *Psychological Bulletin*. **108**(2): 171–94.

19 *Collins Concise Dictionary* (2003) HarperCollins Publishers, Glasgow.

20 Giddens A (1976) *New Rules of Sociological Method*. Hutchinson, London.

21 Handy C (1995) The virtual organization. In: DS Pugh (ed) *Organization Theory*. Penguin Books, London.

22 Nadler DA and Tushman ML (1992) Designing organizations that have good fit: a framework for understanding new architectures. In: M Gerstein, D Nadler and R Shaw (ed) *Organization Architecture*. Jossey-Bass, San Francisco.

23 Peters T and Waterman RH (1982) *In Search of Excellence: lessons from America's best-run companies*. Harper Collins, London.

24 Grindle ME and Hilderbrand ME (1995) Sustainable capacity in the public sector: what can be done? *Public Administration and Development*. **15**: 441–63.

25 Fowler A (1997) *Striking a Balance: a guide to enhancing the effectiveness of non-governmental organisations in international development*. Earthscan, London.

26 Mintzberg H (1983) *Structure in Fives: designing effective organisations*. Prentice Hall International, New Jersey.

27 Dawson S (1996) *Analysing Organisations* (3e). Macmillan Business, London.

28 Crozier M (1964) *The Bureaucratic Phenomenon*. Tavistock, London.

29 Conner DR (1992) *Managing at the Speed of Change*. New York: Villard Books.

30 Maynard A (2005) Competition in health care: what does it mean for nurse managers? *Journal of Nursing Management*. **13**(5): 403–10.

31 Kaplan A (2000) Capacity Building: shifting the paradigms of practice. *Development in Practice*. **10**(3): 517–26.

32 Zairi M and Jarrar YF (2001) Measuring organizational effectiveness in the NHS: management style and structure best practices. *Total Quality Management*. **12**(7&8): 882–9.

33   Gilson L (2002) Trust and development of health care as a social institution. University of Witwatersrand and Health Economics and Financing Programme, Johannesburg.

34   Grindle ME and Hilderbrand ME (1995) Sustainable capacity in the public sector: what can be done? *Public Administration and Development.* **15**: 441–63.

35   Organ DW (1988) *Organizational Citizenship Behavior: the good soldier syndrome.* Lexington Books, Lexington, MA.

36   O'Reilly C and Chatman J (1986) Organisational commitment and psychological attachment: the effects of compliance, identification and internalization on prosocial behaviour. *Journal of Applied Psychology.* **71**(3): 492–9.

37   Parkinson B (1995) *Ideas and Realities of Emotion.* Routledge, London.

38   NHS Plan (2002) Human Resources in the NHS Plan. April 2002. Department of Health, London. www.dh.gov.uk/assetRoot/04/05/58/66/04055866.pdf

39   Osborne S (2002) Vacant Possession. *Health Service Journal.* **9 January**: 24–5.

40   Weston D and Welch A (2003) Recruitment campaign reflects diversity. *Health Service Journal.* **1 May**: 10, 30.

41   Hoban V (2003) How to . . . communicate better with your colleagues. *Nursing Times.* **99**(7): 64–5.

42   Mackintosh M (1981) Gender and economics, the sexual division of labour and the subordination of women. In: K Young, C Wolkowitz and R McCullagh (ed) *Of Marriage and the Market: women's subordination in international perspective.* CSE Books, London.

43   Moore HL (1994) *A Passion for Difference: essays in anthropology and gender.* Blackwell Publishers Ltd, Oxford.

44   Meyer JP and Allen NJ (1997) *Commitment in the Workplace: theory, research and application.* SAGE, London.

45   Mobley WH, Griffeth RW, Hand HH *et al.* (1978) Review and conceptual analysis of the employee turnover process. *Psychological Bulletin.* **86**: 493–552.

46   Bluedorn AC (1982) The theories of turnover: Causes, effects and meaning. In: SW Bacharach (ed), *Perspectives in Organizational Sociology: theory and research*, Vol. 1. JAI Press, New York.

47   Lee TW Mitchell TR Holton BC *et al.* (1999) The unfolding model of voluntary turnover: a replication and extension. *Academy of Management Journal.* **42**(4): 450–62.

48   Peters LH, Bhagat RS and O'Connor EJ (1981) An examination of the independent and joint contributions of organizational commitment and job satisfaction on employee intentions to quit. *Group & Organization Management.* **6**(1): 73–84.

49   Naumann E (1993) Antecedents and consequences of satisfaction and commitment. *Group & Organization Management.* **18**(2): 153–88.

50   Larwood L, Wright TA Desrochers A *et al.* (1998) Extending latent role and psychological contract theories to predict intent to turnover and politics. *Business Organizations Group & Organization Management.* **23**(2): 100–23.

51 Hall C (2005) Crisis looms as foreign nurses quit the NHS. *Daily Telegraph.* **18 May.** www.telegraph.co.uk/core/Content/displayPrintable.jhtml;sessionid=QSTIDSC.

52 Buchan J, Jobanputra R and Gough P (2005) Should I stay or should I go? A survey from the Kings Fund and RCN. *Nursing Standard.* **19**(36): 14–16.

CHAPTER 9

Contributing: managing diversity

The current management definition of diversity emphasises the demographic, surface-level differences (for example age, gender, ethnicity, occupation) within a workforce. The diverse backgrounds of individuals, compounded by the 'work culture' from where they have come, influences the way people communicate and behave in work settings. For example, in some 'cultural settings' it is generally more common for employees to accept authority, while elsewhere individuals tend to be more articulate and confrontational. Some cultures are people-orientated, requiring a lengthy introduction before getting down to business, while for others this seems a waste of time. These underlying beliefs have implications for management in organisations and they have implications for the integration of individuals who are used to functioning in a distinctly different set of norms.[1-4] Diversity has advantages as well as disadvantages when it comes to the productivity of the work team and individual contribution towards overall organisational effectiveness and capacity. Thus understanding of diversity can be seen as a key to integrating migrants, as explained by this 44-year-old female nurse from the Congo:

> The problem is to prepare the mentor or the ward manager to get used to work with nurses from overseas and try to understand that the different way in working is different and help them to integrate in society.

Human resource management involves getting work done through the co-ordinated efforts of others and managers are not only judged by their own performance, but also by the contributions made by their staff. Where employees reflect a wide range of diverse backgrounds, naturally attention should be paid to the management of diversity.

First, issues associated with the positive expression of diversity related to migrant nurses are presented and second, those issues linked to problems with diversity management are highlighted.

Positive expressions of diversity management

As analysis of the day-to-day relationships between migrant nurses and ward managers, nursing sisters or mentors in Chapter 5 shows that these relationships are affected by understanding the individual differences in culture, ethnicity and personal journey. The organisational framework for the way diversity is managed is expressed in written policies and procedures developed by departmental managers, such as 'human resource managers', 'managers of diversity' or 'managers of clinical services'.

Mintzberg's[5] criteria for an effective organisation show that there is no shortcut to nurturing individual employees when an organisation wants to achieve its objectives: '... releasing individual capabilities, values individual contribution ... and looks out for employee well-being, thus nurturing trust and commitment.'

Where a workforce is diverse, it requires managers to pay more attention to issues of equality in access to support and resources, communication and individual respect. Successful management of diversity reflects in positive work-related emotions and also an increased intention of migrant nurses to want to stay with the organisation. Generally migrant nurses are motivated to do their best if they feel supported and treated fairly by their managers, as expressed by a male nurse from the Middle East:

> They tried to support me as much as they can – I will return that and do what I can. It is a general attitude: if they are respecting me, why not stay with them?

This causality could also run the other way and managers should treat those internationally qualified nurses who appear highly motivated favourably and support them during their integration by offering open, two-way communication and respect.

Migrant nurses perceive successful diversity management through interpersonal attitudes and through practical interventions:

- managers welcoming all facets of diversity among their workforce
- managers seeking to understand the newcomers
- managers revealing openness to change
- managers implementing successful communication procedures among nurses who differ in ethnicity and professional status – for example through regular staff meetings providing a forum to discuss practice
- managing such staff meetings in a consultative manner which gives all, including newcomers, freedom to express their points of view
- managers encouraging and facilitating fair and equal professional career development by encouraging participation in training and study days even if there is a shortage in staff

- rewarding and promoting migrant nurses fairly in comparison to British-trained nurses
- managing people with dissimilar career ambitions and different personal commitments in a constructive manner whereby individuals respect each other's differences.

Newcomers appreciate being treated in a fair and equal manner, as this male nurse from Pakistan points out:

> The hospital arranges study days, and during study days they count our hours as a full-time work and they help us to learn the things. They have to pay for someone to go to the ward and also they pay for the class. So it's a very good thing.

During a follow-up interview the same nurse was working effectively in theatre care in the same hospital that supported his supervision period. He therefore stayed with the organisation, reciprocating the investment that was made in him. He had settled into the British approaches to nursing, which differed considerably from Pakistan where he had worked before. Moreover, he continues to learn about the different types of surgery, thereby enhancing his skills and contributing to capacity as a result of his managers treating him equally and giving him support during his integration and career development.

Investment in individuals' career development is key in motivating individuals' commitment to the organisation, but it also offers financial benefits with promotion opportunities and increased salaries. Therefore offering promotion opportunities is not only directly linked to intrinsic work-related motivation, such as increased job satisfaction and a boost in self-confidence and self worth; there is also a direct association with extrinsic benefits in the form of a rise in salary. Moreover, migrant nurses feel psychologically equal, accepted and part of the wider healthcare system as a result of organisational investment into their careers, as one of the nurse informants mentioned:

> I am doing now a D-grade development programme. In a few months my manager will promote me from D grade to E grade. That will be better not only financially, but also psychologically.

Even though a manager may approve of further training activities for internationally qualified nurses, these have to be supported by colleagues at the workplace, as they have to cover for the individual during their study leave. Equality in accessing professional development therefore depends on relationships at work, not just organisational guidelines or managers' good intentions. Thus managing diversity is about more than cross-cultural issues. It also includes managing individuals with different ambitions and attitudes to work. An experienced nurse from Rwanda remarked on this by saying:

I have a study day on Mondays and my manager supports me. The training is exciting, but I found that the problem is with the other nurses: sometimes they are the trouble-makers. They don't like colleagues going on study days. They don't want to go themselves, they want to work, but not study. So, they don't understand others going on study days.

While most NHS trusts provide study days, courses, development programmes and in some cases support for university degrees, not all newcomers feel that these are accessible to them due to resistance within the wider work team. The following statement reflects the gap between what is promised and what is actually delivered to some of the nurses directly recruited from the Philippines:

The Trust is supportive, but the ward managers are the hindrance to our growth, as they don't give us the opportunities announced to us.

A promotion strategy, which considers previous, non-British nursing experience, is one way of demonstrating equality within diversity, as it shows that migrant nurses are not just recruited to fill vacancies but are viewed as individuals with individual professional backgrounds and career aspirations. One manager outlines how this can be implemented in practice:

We pay them a grade-C while they are doing their supervised practice course. A lot of these nurses are very experienced with lots of experience of working overseas and we put them in an area where they have previous experience, so they get developed quicker. For example, if they have ITU experience in their country, part of our criteria here for that grade is that they have the NB 100 and we maintain consistency in that, but that doesn't mean that they wouldn't be supported to do that straight away.

Implementing such a competency-based career development scheme allows the specialist nurses and those with experience to progress quicker. There is the risk, however, that this causes conflict between newly arrived and long-serving staff who have not been promoted. It is therefore important for the whole team to understand and embrace the promotion process in order to prevent in- and out-group behaviour and resentments. Once implemented thoughtfully, competency-based promotion schemes could strengthen commitment among the workgroup.

Even though it needs to be recognised that offering promotion opportunities is not a guarantee that individuals will stay with the organisation, not offering any career development opportunities or offering them in a discriminatory way definitely contributes to high attrition rates.

While diversity management is not exclusive to cross-cultural issues or newcomers to the organisation, cultural diversity and variations of cultural understanding within certain ethnic groups are certainly factors that managers and other team members need to learn to appreciate in order to achieve equality. Cultural understanding among the staff can benefit the organisation by allowing ideas and suggestions to flow forth more unconditionally. Thereby every team member can contribute and this can lead to some truly innovative ideas.

As was shown above, having a diverse team can make some patients feel more comfortable and understood. While there may be dangers of miscommunication, the following example shows that cross-cultural communication can equally be effective and there are dangers in cultural stereotyping. Cultural consideration may not necessarily make any difference to the clinical care a patient receives, but as it is a good example of respect, it should make a contribution to overall patient well-being, as well as educating colleagues of the importance of cultural gestures. An NHS diversity manager gave the following example:

> A nurse from India was being offered a placement on the HIV unit and her initial reaction was: 'No, I don't want to do that.' HIV is very much a taboo subject in India. She still did it despite that first reluctance and really enjoyed it. Talking to her, she felt that because of her Asian background she could understand the Asian patients better. One example was a patient whom they had to take for an examination and they wheeled him head first out of the room and she stopped them and said, 'No, you can't do this, you have to turn it around. It is really important, if you wheel patients head first it means that they are going to die.'

Open discussion of some cross-cultural concerns and policies, which also relate to differences in nursing ethic, can easily be part of the induction programme early on in the integration process. Without putting a value on better or worse practices, such open discussions can aid learning from each other and thus open up a two-way-communication and learning process.

For example, some African migrant nurses may have been used to operating autonomously while others from Eastern Europe may have been used to depending entirely on doctors' orders. For all, getting used to the boundaries, challenges and responsibilities in the UK healthcare system requires a change in behaviour. Yet UK-trained nurses can easily get impatient with newcomers if they do not understand their previous professional ways of carrying out their nursing function. Equally, UK-trained nurses of minority ethnic origin may have further facets of diversity to add, showing that diversity management relates not just to migration. One diversity manager reported:

> So quite regularly we put on a programme on 'ethnicity'. But we also acknowledge that our staff are from a variety of countries, not only the adaptation staff – there are people who have been born here, but are from different origins.

While such workshops and seminars about issues related to diversity and ethnicity may be one step in the right direction, if these discussions do not form part of day-to-day working life, they will make little difference to true interpersonal understanding. Diversity management needs to become an integral part of any workforce representing differences in culture, religion, age, gender, ethnicity, educational level, nationality or employment status and working arrangements.

The issue of diversity management highlights the interrelation of management policies, career development and the effects on overall organisational cohesion and capacity. Diversity is about more than implementing procedures; it is about relationships at work, with all members of work teams, including the newcomers, developing a deeper understanding of multiple identities and how to support individual capabilities.

Problems associated with diversity management

A lack of understanding of diversity issues, including some of the multiple pressures and migration-related issues migrant nurses face, can create serious problems related to workgroup cohesion, organisational commitment and job satisfaction, ultimately affecting nurse retention. These are some of the areas where problems can occur:

- working shifts or long days affects all groups of nurses, but it can create particular problems for migrant nurses, such as refugees who need to present themselves in person at specific times in order to sort out their personal lives
- not having an awareness of and sensitivity to the pressures on the stranger, the migrant
- not being motivated to integrate individuals with diverse backgrounds
- being prejudiced towards newcomers and discriminating against them either overtly or hidden
- not embracing the newcomers skills and professional experience
- not offering any encouragement or affirmation
- not acknowledging the migrant's professional or religious background
- while migrant nurses have to get used to the NHS or 'British' way of doing things, this should not imply that their previous way of operating is inferior. 'I want you to know, we are not in your country' is not an attitude that reflects inclusion
- not promoting migrant nurses or other nurses from minority groups into senior positions.

Some of these issues need to be addressed in very practical ways, such as providing nurses with a satisfactory working schedule, and mixing different shift patterns so that nurses do not have to use up their annual leave in order to meet personal and migration-related matters.

Addressing motivational issues among managers and colleagues is more complicated, as illustrated in this comment made by a nurse from Africa:

> The ward manager was not prepared to work with people from other backgrounds. If they were really motivated it would be better.

In addition, being new to the organisation and being a stranger makes it very awkward for some migrant nurses to convince their managers of their capabilities. Not being known can place much pressure on the individual, who may feel anxious to prove their capacity but receive little encouragement or affirmation. One nurse from Ghana reported how this affected her self-esteem and how her professional competence was put into question:

> You could get one or two who still gave you the recognition as a registered nurse, but during the daily activities on the ward it happens that you have to do the junior person's job. I ask myself why should I go through this? I had my full nursing recognition before I came to this country.

Migrant nurses' contributions are not always recognised or valued by their managers or colleagues. At the same time, to be assigned specialised nursing duties can on the one hand affirm capabilities, but on the other hand, if not remunerated appropriately it can at best cause demotivation and at worse present exploitation as these remarks show:

> We are called to work when they are understaffed, but they gave us a workload assigned for a 405 or E-grade, but we are only paid a D-grade.

> I am contributing a lot of work to the group, working an extra mile, but my workgroup doesn't care.

Individuals respond differently to lack of recognition or taxing organisational management, with some feeling gloomy while others enjoy the challenge and persevere. Thus, together with the training and support provided, the personal traits and abilities should not be underestimated and have to be considered in the way individuals are being managed.

For many managers, the added responsibilities that they face when working with a diverse workforce can be equally demanding. Integrating migrants into an existing workforce is a multifaceted process, and establishing the capabilities and working with internationally qualified nurses from a range of different countries can be a complicated, time- and labour-intensive process. In order to make these investments into people worthwhile, managers have to focus on the long-term outcomes in the form of greater motivation, capacity and retention. Again, some find this difficult but are able to overcome the pressures, while others may not be sufficiently prepared for the management of diversity and need more training.

Managers face the difficult task of integrating nurses who were used to working in a different healthcare system and have to bridge the discrepancy between nurses' competencies and the British regulatory nursing framework, as this comment made by an NHS manager makes clear:

> Some of them don't always appreciate that we supervise them for the right reasons: 'I am a qualified nurse, I don't need to do this' – like a child – 'I don't need to do this.' But we have to ensure that they are safe to practise as a registered nurse. The ward is under huge pressure and if you are delegating a task you need to be sure that it is done. Sometimes there are tensions and the biggest one we have had was with drugs. They can't understand that you can't give two Paracetamol unless a registered nurse is there, and that has caused problems because they are so used to giving them, even antibiotics.

This manager seemed exasperated by the migrants' failure to be 'safe to practise' and therefore dismisses them as 'children'. Other managers have used terms such as coming 'from a backward place', 'from a cave' or draw conclusions about individuals' nursing capabilities on the basis of their English accents or the colour of their skin. Clearly such attitudes and lack of verbal control do not contribute to good diversity practices. Instead, despite the multiple pressures on managers, mentors and supervisors, they need to be able to offer some individual support based on flexibility, a willingness to engage with diverse sub-groups of migrants and an ability to assess an individual's skills, voicing constructive criticism where necessary.

Managers also have the difficult task of deciding if a newcomer is going to meet the required standards. Supported by equal opportunities legislation, it is extremely important to be fair and equal in assessing competencies and, where they are not met despite the individual having received additional support, to be seen as procedurally fair when contracts have to be terminated.

Where managers recognise individual needs and support the integration of migrant nurses' capabilities into organisational capacity this makes a clear contribution to positive outcomes for their organisations. In particular, the nurses' intention to stay with the organisation and their reported level of job satisfaction are important indicators of the success of integration strategies and the management of diversity as one aspect of this wider strategy.

References

1   Brown AD (1998) *Organisational Culture*. Prentice Hall, London.

2   Guirdham M (1999) *Communicating Across Cultures*. Macmillan Press Ltd, London.

3 Lewis RD (1996) *When Cultures Collide: managing successfully across cultures*. Nicholas Brealey Publishing Limited, London.

4 Triandis HC (1995) *Individualism & Collectivism*. Westview Press, Oxford.

5 Mintzberg H (1983) *Structure in Fives: designing effective organisations*: Prentice Hall International, New Jersey.

CHAPTER 10

The way forward

This book contributes to existing knowledge by its exploration of the impact of migration and ethnicity on workplace integration, based on individual perceptions of work-related identities, relationships at work, intrinsic and extrinsic motivation, emotional well-being at work, organisational effectiveness and the management of diversity. These employment characteristics are assessed within existing conceptual frameworks.

Contrary to some popular opinions which view migrants as a burden to the country, the findings presented in this book show that migrant nurses are in fact making valuable contributions to British healthcare organisations. The analysis of the migrants' journey towards integration exposes the importance of relational aspects of organisational capacity and the impact of work-related relationships on social inclusion and intrinsic work-related motivation.

The empirical study underpinning some sections of this book set out to explore the integration of migrant nurses, as one sub-group of international migrants, into employment in the British healthcare sector and their contribution to organisational capacity. The interpretation of their stories exposes characteristics of migrants' integration into employment as part of their resettlement into a developed, Western country, thereby not only contributing to the documented range of migrant experiences, but also pointing the way to better managing the processes of integration.

Before outlining the way forward, this chapter presents a summary of the three elements discussed in this book, namely:

1 migrant nurses' motivation
2 their integration and
3 the contribution they make and implications for diversity management

Motivation

International migration and particularly forced migration directly affects the migrants' integration into work – in this instance in Britain, but the same would be the case for any other Western country. The refugee nurses, as one sub-group of migrant nurses, depend on the co-operation of their employers and the Home Office in order to obtain a valid work permit and resolve their legal status to reside in Britain. Unlike voluntary migrants, such as directly recruited internationally qualified nurses, many of the refugee nurses were not prepared to come to Britain and often have nothing to return to. For some of them the lengthy process to decide on their residence status in Britain causes great uncertainty and distress, making it difficult to establish long-term career plans.

Due to personal problems and having to overcome barriers to employment, most nurses who migrate to Britain independently of recruitment agencies do not access work until some years following their arrival. Particularly for refugee nurses, it is not uncommon to take several years to regain sufficient security as regards their personal situation, immigration status, work permit and understanding of the employment process for nurses in Britain to be able to access employment. As a result many of them experience low levels of self-esteem and are lacking self-confidence.

Employers' uncertainty about the asylum process and the documentation involved further hinders migrants' integration, with some employers shying away from employing asylum seekers and refugees. Instead of contributing their skills, some asylum seekers are left to work illegally in unskilled employment for less than the national minimum wage and in unregulated working conditions. Being allowed access to worthwhile employment clearly is an important stepping-stone on their journey to being self-sufficient and rebuilding their lives.

While some newcomers receive support and understanding, others are met with prejudices and discrimination. Prejudices hindering integration are focused on ethnicity or race and perceptions about the quality of nursing qualifications from other countries, rather than on individuals' immigration status. Often colleagues do not understand the wider issues related to being a migrant and indeed few migrants feel comfortable sharing details of their personal stories at work. Consequently, as colleagues often do not know the latter, interactions with and reactions to the migrants' 'otherness' are normally based on physical appearance. This can lead to feelings of isolation, not being understood and thus being excluded. Many facets of prejudice can impinge negatively on equality and hinder migrant nurses' integration in the day-to-day work environment.

As a result of forced migration, it is common for women from Eastern and Central African countries to leave with just their children, not their male partner, who may follow later. Many of these women have to resort to coping strategies which are not reliant on the support of relatives or familiar social structures, but on individual initiative.[1] Acceptable norms for women migrants vary in different regions and also influence subsequent adaptation to life in

Britain. While some female nurses migrate independently, this is unacceptable in the eyes of others.

Jobs in the British healthcare system still reflect a gender division, with women filling the 'caring' posts and men the 'status' ones;[2] furthermore, there is still a division based on ethnicity, with even fewer minority ethnic and Black women in senior positions. Besides, the fluidity of the terms 'ethnicity' and 'race' is too often not reflected in the statistics on employment and residency of individuals from minority ethnic groups in Britain, which aim to categorise individual ethnic identity. Even though insufficient in themselves, legislation and policies are a step in the right direction.

A strong association between integration, constructive relationships and positive work-related feelings form part of the intrinsic motivation to work. Perceived lack of support from supervisors has a similarly far-reaching impact on the individuals' integration and well-being: it causes work-related stress and makes individuals doubt their abilities. Motivation to work has to be a balance between intrinsic motivators (regaining confidence and self-worth) and extrinsic motivators, such as pay, which some of the directly recruited nurses found inadequate.

- Motivation for migration affects individuals' motivation to work as part of their wider attempt to resettle.
- Motivation for and mode of migration affect integration into employment due to complex policy issues related to work permits, professional standards and available support networks.
- Cultural differences in gender norms further complicate integration.
- Colleagues' prejudices towards Black and minority ethnic members of the team are mainly based on physical appearance, not on migration status.
- Additional personal commitments, such as caring for dependants or financial responsibilities, seem to have a positive effect on career and organisational commitment and a negative one on stress.

Migration positively affects:

- individuals' motivation to work
- the migrants' desire to develop professionally
- the migrants' appreciation of supportive and respectful relationships at work.

Some migrant nurses face exclusion when accessing employment in Britain and the following issues are apparent:

- employers' unfamiliarity with immigration and work permit processes
- differences in professional nursing qualifications compared to other countries

- differences in practical day-to-day nursing duties and professional status compared to other countries
- colleagues' prejudices or racist attitudes, which are primarily based on ethnicity, not migration status
- lack of English language ability, which stresses exclusion by marking out different sub-groups of migrant nurses
- differences in culture and gender norms complicating integration
- the experience of negative work-related feelings during early stages of the integration process, such as feelings of isolation, despair, loss of self-worth
- relationships with their supervisors or mentors, with some showing respect towards the stranger while others pass judgement on the migrants' past experience based on them being 'different'
- entering work leads to a process of transition and re-definition of behavioural and contextual norms for the individual.

Even though all sub-groups of migrants lose familiar points of reference and have to adjust to their host country's cultural norms, for refugees the psychological process seems more complex, with no opportunity to return should integration fail.

Integration

The first stepping-stone in the progression towards integration relates to migrant nurses gaining access to a supervision placement. With a shortfall in places, many internationally qualified nurses, particularly those who come to Britain independently of recruitment agencies, have to accept a place in any nursing discipline regardless of their previous speciality or future ambitions. To achieve registration with the Nursing and Midwifery Council as a nurse in Britain is an important milestone on the road to integration. Accomplishing this gives migrant nurses a boost which affects their personal as well as their work-related identity. This is particularly significant among refugee nurses who have limited alternatives.

This summary of migrants' integration focuses largely on relationships at work which not only form important milestones along the journey of integration, but also act as a mediating factor between the individual newcomer and the organisation. For migrant nurses key relationships are with:

1 their colleagues
2 their mentor and
3 other supervisors and managers.

Interpersonal relationships at work are one of the most important motivating or demotivating factors during the migrants' integration process and therefore relationships form an important component in achieving organisational capacity which relies on individual contributions. Relationships at work present one important aspect of intrinsic motivation, as they convey support, acceptance, respect, dignity, but also unfairness or prejudice, thus encouraging or blocking integration into British employment.

Relationships with colleagues show distinctions depending on the status of colleagues, such as the level of their nursing qualification. While many fully registered nurses are reported to be understanding and supportive of migrant nurses, some of the agency nurses may feel, unjustifiably so, more threatened in their job security. Being ignored, bullied or approached with sarcasm by colleagues leads to feelings of isolation and exclusion among the migrants. This is enhanced by verbal cross-cultural communication problems, which can exacerbate existing prejudices.

Relationships with mentors seem to indicate that these are either very positive or quite negative. On the whole there are few balanced reports about this important relationship, which is key to the integration process, as the mentor recommends internationally qualified nurses to be registered with the Nursing and Midwifery Council. Negative reports about mentors include inadequate one-to-one interaction and insufficient time spent with the mentor, with some nurses not having met their mentor at all. Shift patterns and too much pressure on the mentors' time, as well as some not being prepared to work with minority ethnic nurses, complicate this relationship. In some cases where migrants have a demoralising relationship with their mentor, other staff members take on a mentoring role, introducing the nurse to unfamiliar aspects of work. On a positive note, some migrant nurses compliment their mentors for being supportive, putting themselves into their situation and facilitating access to documents and personal development.

Relationships with other supervisors show similar polarities, with relationships either being encouraging, supportive and empowering or distressing and demoralising. Supportive relationships with at least one other member of staff, mostly a senior colleague, ease the migrant nurse's integration and therefore foster identification with and commitment to the organisation, thus also enhancing feelings of job satisfaction and general well-being at work.

Relationships can convey support, acceptance, respect and dignity, but they also produce negative images, such as lack of cross-cultural sensitivity or prejudice. Work-related emotions extend into the personal sphere with positive experiences at work enhancing self-worth with associated feelings of 'happiness', of 'being accepted', 'liked' and 'trusted', all contributing to self-identity. Part of workgroup and organisational identity rests on 'being liked' or being part of an 'in-group'.

The way migrants are met by colleagues either reinforces their strangeness and otherness, leading to exclusion, or encourages their integration as an appreciated equal, despite being different.

- The individual journey of migrant nurses, including refugee nurses, needs to be regarded with respect and trust, so that motivation can result from relationships as well as the tasks themselves, ensuring integration and personal well-being.
- For refugee nurses the integration into work is a fundamental step in rebuilding their lives.
- Relationships at work and in particular the migrant nurse's relationship with the assigned mentor or another supervisor are an important factor in assisting integration by making the newcomer feel welcomed rather than a burden to others.
- Relationships present a bridge between the 'stranger' and the institution.
- Poor relationships convey feelings of inferiority and insecurity.
- Positive relationships convey value and respect.
- The initial introduction of the newcomer to existing team members is important, as positive introductions are associated with positive socialisation.

A range of emotions, influenced by relationships at work, marks the journey towards professional integration. Work-related feelings symbolise a progressive journey towards integration, with negative feelings frequently expressed during the early stages of employment in Britain and positive ones following professional recognition. In the early stages of employment migrant nurses can feel: 'bad', 'hurt', 'suffering', 'discouraged', 'met with hostility or prejudice' and 'excluded as result of language problems'. Following registration with the Nursing and Midwifery Council, migrant nurses commonly experience more positive work-related emotions, such as feeling 'confident', 'happier', 'liked' and 'trusted'.

- Work-related emotions can act as an indicator of successful integration.
- Intrinsic motivation is linked to individual and work-related identities and encouraged by supportive relationships at work.
- Perceptions of fairness or support are aspects of intrinsic motivation and a range of human needs are met through successful employment experiences.

Generally, where individuals' commitment to the profession is more important to them than commitment to the organisation, employees may choose to change employers in order to advance their career. At the same time as being committed to career development, migrant nurses who have come to Britain independently also express great loyalty to the organisation that supports their supervision. This is partly due to the fact that they are already settled.

Personal identities, such as caring responsibilities for dependants or financial responsibilities outside Britain, seem to be positively relate to the migrant nurses' commitment to the organisation and to their overall well-being at work. Even though these types of commitment may be based on a continued need to be employed in order to meet financial burdens, there is no indication that these nurses are unhappy at work or exercised less effort.

Contribution and diversity management

For some of the migrant nurses, unfamiliar rules seem to undermine their professional confidence, making it difficult to contribute, sometimes out of fear of litigation. But with gradual integration, feelings of confidence return, accompanied by feelings of being trusted by patients and colleagues. Examples of individual contributions include covering for colleagues, sharing past experience, being supportive and caring towards team members, contributing cultural and language knowledge to help patients and being engaged in organisational citizenship behaviour. The experiences of the day-to-day working lives of migrant nurses show that the managers' attitude towards them and a general willingness to explore new ways of working are key precursors to the contribution of capabilities towards organisational capacity.

Some managers compliment migrant nurses on their maturity, strong motivation and emotional strength, but they also indicate that direct international recruitment is only a short-term answer to capacity problems, whereas the integration of migrant nurses already living in Britain is a favourable alternative. Yet some managers may still be apprehensive of proactively supporting internationally qualified nurses who had come to Britain independently of recruitment agencies.

With varying concepts of organisational effectiveness, which may incorporate 'in-role' or 'extra-role' performance, such as organisational citizenship behaviour, the causality of work-related commitment having a direct positive effect on overall organisational performance is so far not empirically clear. Moreover, a 'sense of belonging' and 'of identification' can affect job satisfaction which is positively related to extra-role performance. However, claims that 'happy workers' work harder overall seem misconceived, as they oversimplify the argument.[3] Thus a 'happy worker' can make a positive contribution to the capacity of the workgroup by contributing to the creation of a positive, productive atmosphere. Yet job satisfaction is viewed as the fit between expectations and actual experiences at work and employees who are motivated seem more prepared to contribute to the organisation and make suggestions for improvement.[4]

Policy implementation, such as equal opportunities, together with the experiences of working relationships with supervisors, managers and the work team contribute to a working atmosphere in which newcomers feel able to identify with British nursing approaches and gain confidence to contribute skills and knowledge. Work-related identities fostered through constructive management support, viewing diversity as an asset, can translate into individual nurses committing to the workgroup and/or the organisation and experiencing positive work-related feelings.

To address inequalities in the way Black and minority ethnic employees are treated at work, equal opportunities policies, even though an important step in the right direction, are insufficient in themselves, as in some cases day-to-day practices indicate exclusion. Like many British-trained nurses, few migrant nurses would resort to the official complaints procedures or consult members of the human resource teams when they encounter difficulties. Thus the implementation of such policies requires the thoughtfulness and willingness of individuals in managerial positions to be fair and overcome their own prejudices. Even though racism is not always explicit, it can still be inherent in the way some individuals exclude others on the basis of ethnicity in everyday working life. Demographic variables, such as organisational statistics on diversity, cannot replace the psychological processes that individuals have to go through in order to integrate.[5] It takes time and effort to establish new identities on levels that go deeper than skin colour.

It also has to be recognised that some approaches to equal opportunities implementation can lead to tensions, with existing organisational culture and individual attitudes if nurses are promoted not on the basis of tenure, as was done in the past, but on the basis of an individual's capabilities – regardless of his or her ethnicity or migration status. Morris[6] refers to such considerations, which are based on a view of integration, as a two-way process, in which strangers are appreciated for who they are, despite being different. While agreeing with this view, this book asserts the complications related to implementing such values in practice.

- There are crossing points between personal identities, skills and ambitions and aspects of workplace identity, opportunities and management style.
- Processes such as team building and work-related communication are influenced by management style and policies and can be improved.
- Migrant nurses appreciate managers trying to put themselves into their shoes, offering individual support if required, expressing respect and empathy towards the individuality of migrant nurses, making them feel appreciated and valued.
- Because of their dedication to the organisation that supports their access to employment and because of their strong professional identity a high proportion of migrant nurses are determined to develop their careers.
- Differing cultural patterns are reflected in explicit and implicit norms as well as the behaviours and values within organisations. For some, the procedures in the NHS can seem inflexible and bureaucratic in stark contrast to their past experience, making it difficult to contribute effectively at the beginning of their integration period.

- This can be minimised through diversity training for staff or attention being paid to diversity issues during the induction process.
- Benefits of successful integration are job satisfaction for the individual and their intention to stay with the organisation, thereby addressing the retention problem in the NHS.
- There is evidence to substantiate the positive effect of job satisfaction and positive work-related emotions on individuals' willingness to make a contribution to the wider organisational objectives.

Migrant nurses are adding insightfulness and maturity to existing work teams through:

- their personal stories
- their past clinical experience
- their ability to speak languages shared by some Black and minority ethnic patients
- their understanding of non-British cultures
- their personal strengths, including maturity, emotional strength, resilience to cope under pressure and leadership abilities.

The previous chapters make clear that the employment of minority ethnic nurses and particularly migrant nurses needs to be carefully managed in order to achieve successful integration. Management practices that consider and value diversity among individuals and encourage the individual migrant nurse, not only benefit them through experienced job satisfaction, but also the organisation, as nurses are inclined to stay with the organisation or profession. The following are some of the management issues:

- the employment of migrant nurses who migrate independently to Britain add considerable diversity to work teams and managers need to be aware of the impact on group relationships
- to motivate members of a diverse work team, quality time needs to be invested in communication structures in order to avoid misunderstandings and increase feelings of mutual acceptance
- sensitive and respectful one-to-one communication is a key area of concern to the nurses.

Successful diversity management goes beyond equal opportunities policies and reflects in day-to-day relationships and procedural fairness in the way migrant nurses are treated in comparison to British-trained nurses. Once the management of individuals who are different is addressed, the successful management of diversity contributes to addressing the following economic issues which are currently of concern to healthcare providers in Britain.

- The employment of Black and minority ethnic nurses makes NHS trusts in London more reflective of the community they are serving.
- The employment of migrant nurses who migrated independently contribute to addressing recruitment issues and save on agency costs.
- The employment of this sub-group of migrant nurses contributes to addressing retention issues in the NHS as many independent migrants both show a desire to stay with the organisation that supports their integration and also have few plans to leave Britain.

This book contributes to existing knowledge by showing that positive socialisation during the early stages of the employment relationship and open, respectful communication structures can break down barriers and prejudices among demographically different individuals. Within a supportive environment, one-to-one encounters between ethnically and culturally different individuals highlight deeper-level commonalities, which are often not explored, as most people spontaneously act upon surface-level differences, such as age, skin colour or dress code.

Thus people-centred management is fundamental to capacity building. Where human interactions are managed with consideration for individual needs, individual newcomers can feel empowered and experience greater motivation to contribute at work. In turn the organisation benefits through nurses positively interacting with other members of the work team, showing engagement with work and a desire for professional development.

Table 10.1 summarises the findings on features of workplace integration as seen from the perspectives of the individual migrant nurse and then the organisational managers. This provides an overview in relation to sub-groups of internationally qualified nurses.

The influence of personal identities on experiences of the workplace, which are central to individual contributions to organisational capacity, is summarised in Figure 10.1. Aspects of personal identities affect how managers' act and how the working environment is experienced and evaluated. Mediated by relationships and emotions at work, this has implications for the individual as well as for the organisation.

Exclusion or inclusion in employment

Since the influx of migrants from Commonwealth countries after World War II, barriers to their integration, such as prejudices and racism have become more explicit in management frameworks. Such policies, however, are not always effective in addressing individual attitudes.

This book makes a key contribution to the concept of social exclusion by showing that exclusion, based on personal characteristics, more commonly

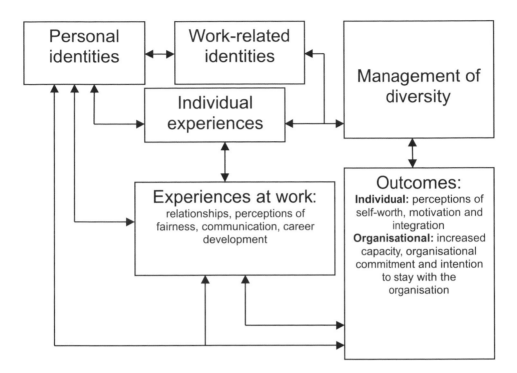

Figure 10.1 Workplace experiences as bridge or barrier to contribution.

results from ethnic characteristics than from the individual migration journey. While individuals' motivations to migrate can be unclear, there are boundaries between migration, ethnicity and culture. Ethnicity is commonly defined by physical features and relates to surface-level diversity, while the migration experience is a personal story, often withheld within the employment context. Yet the journey of integration into employment forms a key aspect of resettlement.

Therefore being different and perceived as a 'stranger' by the majority culture is primarily based on external characteristics of individuals and can lead to prejudices. Such prejudices are based on preconceived ideas related to cultural stereotyping and set ideas of ethnicities. On the part of the migrant, feeling excluded in such a way prohibits any further interpersonal contact and sharing of 'self' with others. Social exclusion at work substantiates a 'them' and 'us' approach which disagrees with constructive management processes aiming at group cohesion, inclusion, equality and effectiveness.

Through sharing personal stories, meaningful one-to-one encounters emerge and the stranger becomes a person who becomes included as shared personal experiences bridge differences created by surface-level diversity. Labelling individuals has social consequences at work, yet as a result of person-to-person contact between the newcomer, the migrant and colleagues or supervisors,

Table 10.1 Stages and measures of integration into employment

Groups of migrant nurses	Access to healthcare employment in Britain	The employment of migrant nurses		
		Motivation	Integration	Contribution
All migrant nurses who have migrated to Britain independently	• English language requirement (IELTS test) • Learning about the British healthcare system, regulatory bodies (NMC), government policies (DH) • Lack of information about the procedures and process of applying for registration with the NMC • Personal issues, family commitments, housing, especially in London • Cultural and psychological issues • Danger of abuse by unregulated healthcare employers • Lack of awareness of rights in Britain • Delays in applications for registration being processed • Lack of supervision placements	Exclusion due to differences: • differences in qualifications • differences in nursing ethic norms • differences in gender norms • lack of language proficiency Exclusion due to experience of relationships: • prejudices among lesser qualified colleagues, based on ethnicity • racism expressed by a few colleagues and supervisors Additional pressures: • caring responsibilities, especially female migrants • isolation from family and support network	Relationships at work as motivating factor – positive emotions: • mentor or supervisor very helpful • offer of individual support • expression of interest in the personal story • offer of career development, promotion • job satisfaction, feeling happy Relationships at work as demotivating negative emotions: • breakdown of the relationship with the mentor • lack of support or respect • lack of cross-cultural management experience • miscommunication • feelings of gloom and stress.	Management of diversity – barriers or encouragements to integration: • lack of understanding of diversity management • lack of attention paid to workgroup socialisation • prejudices based on surface-level diversity • perceived unfairness regarding length of supervision period • procedural fairness in the way equal opportunities are implemented • value and respect of previous professional experience Contributions to capacity: • language ability • understanding of non-British cultures • improving patient care
Directly internationally recruited migrant nurses	• Involvement of recruitment agency • Some type of employment guaranteed	• Establish independent roots, if a group of migrant nurses were recruited together to work in the same organisation	• Supervision period predetermined • Mutual support, as most arrive in groups of colleagues, recruited simultaneously	• Introduction and supervision period pre-planned • Lack of consideration of nurses' desires as to career development

Additional issues faced by refugee nurses	• Uncertainty related to immigration status • Lack of documents to prove past training, qualifications and work experience – affecting supervision placement • Difficulty in obtaining references • Issues related to pre- and in-flight experiences • Permanence of integration	• Personal problems related to migration identity • Need for additional support, flight-interrupted employment • Employers' unfamiliarity with immigration procedures and documentation • Prejudices based on wrong understanding of asylum seekers	• Due to experienced loss, particular to forced migration, the range of experienced feelings can potentially be more far-reaching, reflecting loss	• Refugee nurses personal adaptability to stress at work reported by a few managers • Gratitude towards employing organisations as work expressed important stepping-stone within wider integration, expressed by some refugee nurses

Measures of successful integration related to research objectives

Individual measures of successful integration through personal identity and personal aspects of organisational effectiveness	• A work environment that values women, employees from minority ethnic groups and migrants, treating them fairly with regard to recruitment, management and promotion • Appreciation of migration experience • Individual support from supervisors • Positive efforts to enhance communication among colleagues through careful team building and socialisation	• High commitment to the organisation as result of positive organisational identification • More positive (happiness) than negative (stress and gloom) work-related feelings, related to well-being at work • Increased self confidence and self-worth • Relationships at work which convey acceptance, support, respect and dignity • Balance of extrinsic and intrinsic motivational factors	• Personal job satisfaction which contributes to overall well-being, providing the basis from which to contribute • Promotion opportunities and support for career development • Constructive management of diverse teams • Implementation of equal opportunities reflected in procedural fairness • Supportive supervisor taking personal circumstances into account • Feeling equal and accepted, thus integrated

Table 10.1 *(continued)*

Groups of migrant nurses

	The employment of migrant nurses		
	Motivation	*Integration*	*Contribution*
Organisational measures of successful integration through organisational capacity building	• Cohesion among diverse workgroups • Appreciation of individual capabilities • Diversity reflecting the local community, enhancing credibility among the public and patients • Cultural understanding by nurses improve patient well-being	• High levels of effective commitment to the workgroup and organisation • Staff exercising organisational citizenship behaviour • Staff feeling motivated to work reflecting in work effectiveness • Effective communication among diverse team members	• Capacity reflected in the retention of nurses who gain registration in Britain • Nurses making positive contribution to the organisation, contributing to organisational objectives • Intention to stay with the organisation • Intention to apply past experience on behalf of the organisation • Being able to exercise innovation • Valuing and integration of past professional experience

preconceived ideas of people take on a new significance, stressing the positive impact of constructive work-related relationships on social inclusion. Through supportive relationships at work the newcomer's face becomes a person, an individual with feelings and identities, able to integrate and contribute as a result of being welcomed.

Existing studies confirm only parts of this linkage, with Perryman et al.[7] showing that a supportive relationship with the line manager is a principal agent in achieving job satisfaction. Arnold et al.[8] state that perceived lack of consideration by the boss towards employees caused job pressure and work-related stress. Due to the amount of time spend at work, work-related relationships and the social support network at work contribute to individual well-being and ease job strain.

With relational, interpersonal factors shaping team effectiveness, friction among some groups of colleagues raises concerns about the effectiveness of multicultural work teams. Staff can generally feel demotivated if their work-group is not cohesive, with colleagues being hostile or unsupportive towards each other, including newcomers. This stresses the role that managers have to play in proactively shaping the integration process of diverse work teams. A challenge to organisational managers is to sustain congruence between different individuals' personal identities and organisational aspects in order for employees to experience job satisfaction and motivation and for the organisation to achieve its objectives. The individual nurse's relationship with the supervisor is key in this process, as supervisors are able to identify individual strengths and are also able to ease integration of the newcomer.

In occupations relying on interpersonal contact, such as nursing, effectiveness cannot be measured solely in numerical terms, it needs to take intrinsic work-related motivation into account by noting the contribution of relationships at work to create a positive atmosphere, valuing diversity among individuals. Therefore recruitment strategies should aim not just at increasing nursing numbers but also at increasing diversity, with its related responsibilities for managers. Thus it appears essential to identify some of the motivating factors that are important to keep migrant nurses not only engaged in their profession but also assist their integration to progress from being a stranger to becoming part of an in-group. If such a concept applies to nurses, the same principles could also be applicable to other occupations.

Existing *gender norms* in Britain contrast with those with which migrants are familiar and affect their integration into the workplace. Even though worldwide the majority of nurses are female, it is documented in existing studies that the number of Black and minority ethnic females in leadership positions is comparatively small. This confirms Davies,[9] who said that nursing is viewed commonly as an extension of women's caring role at home, one that is undervalued. However, there are concerns that existing gender differences in British employment may make it doubly difficult for female nurses from Black and minority ethnic backgrounds to progress in their careers, as for them gender discrimination can be compounded by racial discrimination. Existing empirical studies show evidence that female employees are disadvantaged with regard to promotion into more prestigious and better-paid positions compared to males ones.[10] A limitation on promotion opportunities would have serious consequences for the intrinsic motivation of migrant nurses, reinforcing existing retention and effectiveness problems for NHS organisations.

Refugees as one sub-group of international migrants get categorised together with other groups of independent migrants who came to Britain for economic, career or family-related reasons. Since the Geneva Convention is difficult to implement and does not define the term 'persecution' clearly, what constitutes a refugee needs to be revisited. The European Union produced a joint position 96/196/JHA on the harmonised definition of the term 'refugee' in Article 1 of the Geneva Convention of 28 July 1951 relating to the status of refugees.[11] The distinction between 'forced migration' and other motives to come to Britain offers only a crude differentiation, but one with far-reaching practical consequences. Closer co-operation between employers and the Home Office is required to review the existing process. Regulations for applications for asylum are contained in the Immigration and Asylum Act 1999 and the Nationality, Immigration and Asylum Act 2002. Should an asylum seeker be refused asylum there is a right to appeal. In addition to a right to appeal for asylum, it may be possible for immigrants to be granted 'humanitarian protection' (previously known as exceptional Leave to Remain) and to remain in the country for a limited period.

The process of seeking a permanent immigration status adds to the complications faced by migrants upon arrival in Britain. Most refugees from developing countries usually travel to a neighbouring country, in hope of return to their homes. It is rare for them to move on and then be granted asylum in a Western country. UNHCR-led resettlement programmes may provide an alternative for refugees to illegal migration to Britain. Currently the UNHCR has a quota of resettling 100 000 refugees into mainly Western countries; however, only a quarter of this is actually being used.

There seems to be conceptual confusion about the term 'integration' as used by the Home Office, as objectives are unclear and it is difficult to measure the success of integration. Structural government-led forces appear to include minority groups into what is viewed as mainstream society. Such approaches are often based on the expectation that the stranger will take on board common customs, traditions and ways of life. Policies on citizenship training and tests are based on such a model of assimilation. Yet for integration to be successful it has to be seen as a two-way process accompanied by mutual learning and openness to change.

First, attention has to be paid to the socialisation period during the early stages of the journey towards integration into employment. Kanter[12] confirms the importance of giving careful consideration to the initial introduction period when newcomers join an existing team. The achievement of workgroup cohesion among diverse teams can strengthen individual's job satisfaction and commitment to organisational objectives, which form part of the experiences of employment as the journey progresses.

Second, empirical knowledge of diversity in workgroups enhancing innovation, provides a challenge to common organisational practice. Instead of assimilating newcomers into existing practices, mutual sharing of past experiences could contribute to more effective approaches as different ways of achieving objectives are discussed. Individuals feeling valued by supervisors and colleagues strengthens their self-esteem and enables them to have a say. Once the interpersonal relations among diverse team members are managed well, their understanding of each other can contribute to addressing underlying prejudices and release individual capabilities. More attention to the day-to-day management style could create a work environment in which migrants feel motivated, free to contribute and contented to stay long-term. This then contributes to addressing retention problems as a result of poor job satisfaction.

Third, in relation to the concept of social exclusion, the 'other' takes on different meanings for different individuals and ethnic groups. The experiences of resettlement and integration are results of personal characteristics, calling for each newcomer to be treated as an individual. This should warn managers not to group all their 'minority ethnic' employees together, as one seemingly homogenous group. With some attitudes of prejudice and racism being detached from skin colour and ethnicity, promoting equality needs to challenge the concept of viewing individuals from minority ethnic backgrounds as 'victims'.

The extent to which colleagues and supervisors perceive individual diversity as an asset, rather than expecting the stranger to take on board the explicit behaviour of the majority culture, influences integration and subsequent ability to contribute. As a result, management focus should be on both, equal opportunities policies and on training and equipping managers to implement these more effectively as part of workgroup socialisation.

Even though organisations are collecting information on their employees' ethnic background, the fluidity of the 'ethnicity' term is not reflected in such statistics. Liff[13] questions whether diversity initiatives and equal opportunities monitoring can address underlying issues of institutional discrimination based on gender or ethnicity. 'Diversity guidelines' as published by the Royal College of Nursing and Midwifery[14] may therefore not only clash with ongoing practice but also fail to address underlying attitudes. These include the following: making diversity and equality central to strategic business planning, investing in cultural awareness training, understanding the importance of diversity, ensuring compliance with best practice guidelines, monitoring and evaluating the impact of policy and business decisions on equality and diversity.

The effective management of a diverse workforce cannot be monitored through statistical feedback on age, gender, disability, health, sexual orientation, ethnicity and religion. Managers need to look at the relational aspects of the work environment and at feedback that individual nurses give about their day-to-day working experiences, which can offer a valuable picture of the implementation of human resource policies.

This book shows how migrant nurses struggle to integrate as they face institutional hurdles. Unfamiliar nursing tasks and standards, including patients' rights, can be important but also intimidating to newcomers. Even though the unfamiliarity eases throughout the integration process, NHS organisations could benefit from recognising and valuing the experiences and skills among migrant nurses, even where these differ from what NHS managers view as important. A midwife who has learned to work safely without electronic monitoring of the baby's heartbeat will benefit from this technology, which is standard practice in British hospitals, but her clinical skills are probably better developed because she learnt to work safely without the technology. The Refugee Council clearly states that refugees' contributions to employment need to be recognised and some should become role models:

> Positive contributions refugees make in the economic, social and cultural life of Europe must be recognised ... in the sphere of employment refugees must be visible as role models.[15]

In order to develop confidence among new members of the work team, it is important to acknowledge the scope of their previous experience and to treat them with dignity and respect, thus creating an environment of trust in which the nurses can develop and contribute to the overall organisation and its culture. Consequently, it is argued that managers can actively foster the process of migrants contributing their skills to the overall organisation through the building up of trust and the appraisal of individual contributions. This requires managers to be open to change and to invest in finding out how to relate to and motivate individual staff members.

Ultimately individually perceived motivation and well-being need to produce outputs that can be assessed against organisational objectives, such as clinical patient care and working effectively alongside other colleagues. Focusing on aspects of the journey towards integration, the links between management support, work-related emotions, individual capabilities and organisational capacity are strengthened.

In order to encourage nurses into employment, additional practical support considered by some NHS Trusts includes initiatives such as flexible working policies, childcare facilities and the provision of family-friendly accommodation. Some of these policies are supported by employment legislation and to implement them can have a positive impact on employee retention.[16] For example, the Low-Pay Commission sets a national minimum wage and the Employment Bill of 2002[17] gives parents the right to request flexible working arrangements from their employers. The Employment Act 2002 came into effect on 6 April 2003. Section 80 sets out conditions under which an employer is allowed to refuse requests for flexible working.[18]

Reports from working mothers show that the cost of childcare often makes it barely economically worthwhile to work, drawing attention to extrinsic motivation, yet the research linked such family responsibilities to increased work-related commitments.

The continued lack of recognition of migrants' contributions to British organisation remains a key issue, highlighting the importance of more research to strengthen the correlation between immigration status and workgroup cohesion. This is something that has not yet been studied, even though studies have looked at the effects of other aspects of diversity on group processes.[19–24] Further assessment of the journey of progression towards integration would benefit from longitudinal research to determine promotion opportunities and career progression.

In conclusion, integration should not be a process of assimilation, but one of mutual respect with implications for organisational managers and the individual migrant. The integration of migrant nurses into British employment, therefore, relies on a successful merger of organisational objectives and how they are reflected in the day-to-day practice of work-related relationships and individual identities, motivators and capabilities.

Concluding remarks

Tracing the journey of migrant nurses' motivations to come to Britain, their experiences of integrating into healthcare employment and views on the contribution they are making sheds light on migrant working. The exploration of migrant nurses in Britain contributes to the understanding of workplace integration, viewed as a two-way process, and shows that individual motivation can be fostered by constructive cross-cultural management. Thus successful workplace integration first benefits the individual through job satisfaction and individual well-being, something that applies to all groups of employees. Second, in addition to increasing the number of skilled employees, the organisation gains a range of contributions expressed through a diverse workforce, and where migrants come for non-work related reasons, they help address long-term retention problems.

The journey of integration continues to remain a problematic one: while migrants reports contain positive experiences of genuine appreciation of the 'other' they also highlight an urgent need to address underlying attitudes of prejudice which remain, affecting relationships and leading to the exclusion of migrants within the social context of work.

Yasmin Alibhai-Brown, herself a refugee from Uganda, illustrated the difficulties faced by new arrivals in the following comment:

> The reason so many more asylum-seekers and economic migrants are coming here is not because the country is a 'soft touch' but because people can see what immigrants have accomplished here in spite of racism.[25]

However, any obstacles to integration are not just a consequence of racism, but also a lack of awareness or unwillingness among some to notice the plight of strangers. Even though for centuries migrants have set up their homes in Britain, the contributions they have made and continue to make are not always noticed or accredited to them. Emotive views of the current immigration debate do not consider the capabilities that migrants contribute to organisational capacity and society in general.

For centuries the successes of migrants' journeys of integration have left their little-noticed mark in history and it seems fitting to place the current experiences of migrant nurses within this wider historical context, ending with some stories of accomplishment.

- 1685–1700: The Huguenots – their contribution to British society is still evident today. Seven of the 24 founders of the Bank of England were Huguenots. Huguenot midwives and doctors had an impact on healthcare.
- 1933–1939: Jewish refugees – Jewish refugee businessmen were successful in developing interests in the depressed North of the country while in London the textile industry expanded due to their input. Thorn Electrical Industries was established by Sir Jules Thorn, an Austrian Jewish refugee. Doctors and (fewer) nurses had a significant impact on healthcare, for instance in the field of mental healthcare provision.
- 1939–1950: Refugees from communism – 250 000 Polish refugees contributed to building houses, filling labour shortages and laying the foundations of British post-war society.
- 1973–1979: Chileans – Carlos Fortin was among 3000 Chilean refugees and became head of the Institute of Development Studies in Sussex.[26]

The above examples show that, over the centuries, all of these migrants filled gaps in the labour market and made a contribution to British organisations. Greater awareness of the current and historic examples of such contributions made by migrants should ease people's fears of being swamped by strangers. Contrary to public opinion, most migrants, including asylum seekers and refugees, are not asking for pity and looking for handouts, but seek an opportunity to either rebuild or better their lives. The question has to be asked: why do wealthy countries like Britain, which is hosting only 1.98% of the world's refugees,[27] operate a policy that aims to stem migration if some of the poorest countries are left with the burden of massive refugee inflows?

Calls for managed migration aim to tackle abuse of the immigration system by addressing illegal immigration while opening doors to highly skilled migrants. Such approaches seem short-sighted, as much of the country's economy depends on migrant labour. However, this view is not shared by the majority of 15–23 year olds, 58% of whom think that migrants are not making a positive contribution[28] and such attempts of managing migration exclude refugees who have no way of legally accessing safety in Britain.[29]

The book ends with this quote from a leading Anglo-Jewish Rabbi, which challenges not only hostility but also apathy towards the stranger. Speaking from personal experience, this is his petition:

> How you are with the one to whom you owe nothing, that is the grave test . . . I always think that the real offenders at the halfway mark of the century were the bystanders, all those people who let things happen because it didn't affect them directly. I believe that the line our society will take in this matter on how you are to people to whom you owe nothing is a signal. It is a critical signal that we give to our young, and I hope and pray it is a test we shall not fail.
>
> Rabbi Hugo Gryn, Refugee Week, 2002[30]

References

1 Connell RW (1987) *Gender & Power*. Polity Press, Cambridge.

2 Davies C (1995) *Gender and the Professional Predicament in Nursing*. Open University Press, Buckingham.

3 Bassett G (1994) The case against job satisfaction. *Business Horizons*. 7(3): 67.

4 Mullins LJ (2002) Managerial behaviour and effectiveness. In: LJ Mullins (ed) *Management and Organisational Behaviour* (6e). Prentice Hall, London.

5 Lawrence (1997) The black box of organisational demographics. *Organisational Science*. 8: 1–22.

6 Morris L (2002) *Managing Migration, Civic Stratification and Migrants' Rights*. Routledge, London.

7 Perryman S and Robinson D (2003) Down the line. *Health Service Journal*. **17 April**: 26–8.

8 Arnold J, Cooper CL and Robertson IT (1998) *Work Psychology*. Financial Times Publishing, London.

9 Davies C (1995) *Gender and the Professional Predicament in Nursing*. Open University Press, Buckingham.

10 Beishon S, Virdee S and Hagell A (1995) *Nursing in a Multi-ethnic NHS.* Policy Studies Institute, London.

11 European Union (2004) The European Union clarifies what it means by 'refugee'. http://europa.eu.int/comm/justice_home/doc_centre/asylum/refugee/wai/doc_asylum_refugee_en.htm (accessed 20 February 2004).

12 Kanter RM (1977) *Men and Women of the Corporation.* Basic Books, New York.

13 Liff S (1999) Diversity and equal opportunities: room for constructive compromise? *Human Resource Management Journal.* **9**(1): 65–75.

14 RCN (2002) *Diversity Appraisal Resource Guide: helping employers, RCN officers and representatives promote diversity in the workplace.* Royal College of Nursing, London.

15 Gaunt S, Hudson D, Aferiat Y *et al.* (2001) *Good practice guide on the integration of refugees in the European Union.* British Refugee Council, London.

16 Baruch Y and Winkelmann-Gleed A (2002) Multiple commitments: a conceptual framework and empirical investigation in a community health services Trust. *British Journal of Management.* **13**(4): 337–57.

17 Roberts Z and Watkins J (2003) Parental Guidance. *People Management.* **23 January**: 16–17.

18 dti (2004) *Employment Relations. Working Parents. Flexible Working: the right to request and the duty to consider.* www.dti.gov.uk/er/individual/flexwork-pl520.pdf

19 Cox TH, Lobel SA and McLeod PL (1991) Effects of ethnic group cultural differences on cooperative and competitive behaviour on a group task. *Academy of Management Journal.* **34**(4): 827–47.

20 Guirdham M (1999) *Communicating Across Cultures.* Macmillan Press Ltd, London.

21 Kandola R and Fullerton J (1998) *Diversity in Action, Managing the Mosaic* (2e). IPD, London.

22 Larkey LK (1996) Towards a theory of communicative interactions in culturally diverse workgroups. *Academy of Management Review.* **21**(2): 463–91.

23 Iganski P, Mason D, Humphreys A *et al.* (2001) Equal opportunities and positive action in the British National Health Service: some lessons from the recruitment of minority ethnic groups to nursing and midwifery. *Ethnic and Racial Studies.* **24**(2): 294–317.

24 Watson WE, Kumar K and Michaelsen LK (1993) Cultural diversity's impact on interaction process and performance: comparing homogenous and diverse task groups. *Academy of Management Journal.* **36**(3): 590–602.

25 Alibhai-Brown Y (2001) Don't be fooled: the best immigrants are not always the most 'skilled'. *The Independent.* **6 June**. www.independent.co.uk/story.jsp?story=54576.

26 South of England Refugee & Asylum Seeker Consortium (2004) *The Heritage and Contribution of Refugees in the UK.* www.southamptom-city.ac.uk/refugeeweek. 26 February 2004.

27 The Independent (2003) Asylum: the facts. *The Independent.* **23 May**: 1.

28 Greater London Authority (2004) Press Release. www.london.gov.uk/view_press_release. jsp?releaseid=1819. 26 February 2004.

29 Home Office (2003) Effectively managed migration is good for Britain – Home Secretary. 12 November 2003. 309/2003. Home Office, London. www.workingintheuk.gov.uk/working_in_the_uk/en/homepage/news/press/effective ... 5 May 2004.

30 Refugee Week (2002) *Factpack (1) Introduction.*

Index